Praise for *VRx*

"If you have ever wondered what the future of medicine holds, *VRx* is a must-read. It is elegantly written, scientifically accurate, and engaging. Through the voices of patients whose pain, anxiety, and/or suffering have been alleviated by VR, Dr. Spiegel makes the compelling case for VR as a medical treatment for a variety of conditions."

—David C. Rhew, MD, chief medical officer, Microsoft

"*VRx* is an engaging journey into the cutting edge of virtual, augmented, and extended reality. Dr. Spiegel, a leading figure in the field, brilliantly captures the stories and science enabling this emergent field, and the promise of what lies ahead."

—Daniel Kraft, founder and chair, Exponential Medicine, Singularity University

"*VRx* is a compelling, provocative, and highly readable account of the transformative possibilities that VR has inspired across healthcare. Spiegel blends those observations with the critical eye of both a healthcare provider and a scientist, and draws insightful connections between VR and philosophy, neuroscience, meditation, psychedelics, the Information Age, culture, health, and well-being. This is more than just another book about virtual reality. *VRx* asks us to consider the richness of the human experience and the ways that we are challenged to understand it."

—Skip Rizzo, University of Southern California

"If you are curious or concerned about the future of healthcare, then *VRx* is a must-read. It is smart, thoughtful, and informative—not only does Dr. Spiegel provide us with an exciting view of the future of healthcare, he also captivates us by weaving into his narrative a healthy mixture of neuroscience, history, philosophy, and drama."

—Dr. Walter Greenleaf, Stanford University

VR$_X$

How Virtual Therapeutics
Will Revolutionize Medicine

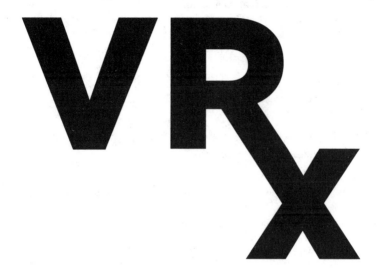

BRENNAN SPIEGEL

BASIC BOOKS

New York

Basic Books
Hachette Book Group
1290 Avenue of the Americas, New York, NY 10104
www.basicbooks.com

Printed in the United States of America

First Edition: October 2020

Published by Basic Books, an imprint of Perseus Books, LLC, a subsidiary of Hachette Book Group, Inc. The Basic Books name and logo is a trademark of the Hachette Book Group.

The Hachette Speakers Bureau provides a wide range of authors for speaking events. To find out more, go to www.hachettespeakersbureau.com or call (866) 376-6591.

The publisher is not responsible for websites (or their content) that are not owned by the publisher.

Print book interior design by Amy Quinn.

All photos courtesy of the author, except the image in the Introduction, which is courtesy of Cedars-Sinai.

Library of Congress Cataloging-in-Publication Data
Names: Spiegel, Brennan, author.
Title: VRx : how virtual therapeutics will revolutionize medicine / Brennan
    Spiegel.
Description: First edition. | New York : Basic Books, 2020. | Includes
    bibliographical references and index.
Identifiers: LCCN 2020001434 | ISBN 9781541699762 (hardcover) | ISBN
    9781541699755 (ebook)
Subjects: LCSH: Virtual reality in medicine. | Virtual reality therapy.
Classification: LCC R859.7.C65 S65 2020 | DDC 610.285—dc23
LC record available at https://lccn.loc.gov/2020001434

ISBNs: 978-1-5416-9976-2 (hardcover), 978-1-5416-9975-5 (ebook)

LSC-C

10 9 8 7 6 5 4 3 2 1

To my wife and children, who make living
in real reality an ever-present joy.

Contents

Author's Note

The following patients were interviewed for this book and graciously allowed their names to appear within their stories: Richard Breton, Danielle Collins, Harmon Clarke, Tom Norris, Robert Jester, and Erin Martucci. The names of other patients were changed and elements of their stories modified to preserve confidentiality.

I have made every effort to write a scientifically accurate book supported by hundreds of citations. However, there are thousands of additional studies that I could not include due to space restrictions. I selected studies that I believe will stand the test of time and relied on randomized controlled trials, when available, to support assertions in the text. Any factual errors in this book are my responsibility; please contact me should you find inaccuracies and I will seek to correct the record.

A Leap of Faith

W HEN VIRTUAL REALITY FIRST TOOK HOLD OF ME, I THOUGHT I was going to die. Walter Greenleaf, a leading virtual reality (VR) scientist from Stanford University, visited my lab at Cedars-Sinai Medical Center in Los Angeles in 2014 with a team of programmers to demonstrate their supercharged tech. They placed a headset over my eyes, and the world disappeared into blackness. It felt as though I were sitting in an unlit cavern awaiting some unwelcome surprise. Suddenly, a bright scene ignited into crisp reality, and I found myself standing outside on a shaky window-washing rig, slowly ascending the side of a fifty-story building. I heard creaking cables and the sound of a steady breeze. I felt the butterflies of anxiety and began swaying in rhythm with the teetering platform beneath my feet.

The rig stopped at the top of the building. I stood looking out upon a downtown cityscape, perched hundreds of feet in the air above a concrete sidewalk. It felt dangerous, even though I was standing in a familiar conference room. My heart was palpitating, nerves were firing, and tendons stiffening. A few seconds passed. I settled in long enough to register the beauty of the scene and note details, like the signage atop buildings, the glint of sunlight reflecting off windows, and traffic patterns in a far-off rotary.

Without warning, the rig's protective railing suddenly detached, plummeting end-over-end and crashing into the street far below. I nearly panicked. Some inner spirit took control of my limbs. I reached back in desperation for the "window" behind me (which was a whiteboard on the conference room wall). I shut my eyes to escape and think. This would all be fine if I could only reason my way through it. My feet knew they were standing on carpet, but how could I get my brain to know this as well?

"Okay, now jump off the platform," said Greenleaf. "Just take one big step into the void."

Not a chance. There was no way I was going to leap off that building. It made no difference that I knew I was in a conference room. This virtual world had commandeered my brain. I was paralyzed with fear.

Reading about VR is like reading about space travel—you might imagine the effortless glide of floating in zero gravity, but until you are in space, well, you're not. Unless you have been inside virtual reality it's hard to imagine how powerful it is. So the next best way to experience it is to watch others try it. Here is one of my patients using VR while suffering from the severe pain of sickle cell anemia. Before taking this picture, he was doubled over from body aches despite taking powerful painkillers. At

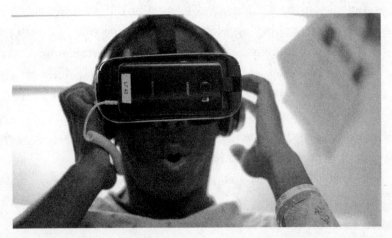

this moment, he is flying in a helicopter over fjords in Iceland. It is hard to tell that he's in pain.*

This book is about why he isn't in pain and what that means for how we treat some of our most pressing health threats.

Perhaps you think that VR is a gaming technology—a toy for pimply, pent-up teens to play first-person shooter games in their parents' basement. You wouldn't be alone. Maybe you have a VR headset for a Sony PlayStation, or you know someone who uses Oculus or Samsung Gear VR to play games in fantasy worlds. Maybe you read *Ready Player One*, the Ernest Cline novel, or saw the movie version, where people become so obsessed with the virtual world that they neglect the real one. Maybe you think of VR as just another addictive screen. And then there's VR pornography . . . that's a whole other story.

People tend to think of VR only in terms of technology that has been brought to the consumer market. They think it's about wearing big goggles. Let me be clear: VR is not about goggles. Today's headsets will cede to tomorrow's VR eyeglasses or contact lenses that are digitally connected to a network of miniaturized body sensors. Future virtual worlds will stimulate not just our vision but all our senses, using smaller, more portable, and less expensive devices. We will be able to travel with VR wherever we go. VR will connect mind and body in a bid to support virtual biofeedback. Wearable activity monitors, heart rate monitors, electroencephalograms, and stress sensors will drive the VR experience in an ever-changing, personalized, immersive experience. These applications will improve the way virtual worlds are created. But they are not what VR really is.

Rather, VR is a way to deliberately and predictably modify how we feel and how we think. It's a platform that connects us to our heart, mind, and body. I mean that literally. VR can be used toward a variety of ends, but I am going to talk specifically about how VR can be used to help us heal in ways that other treatments cannot. As the technology advances, scientists are discovering just how effectively VR alters our perception of

---

* You can watch this video of his VR experience here: www.virtualmedicine.health /patients-using-vr.

reality. We've found that it can manage pain, lower blood pressure, treat eating disorders, and combat anxiety. VR helps deliver babies and enables soldiers to cope with the mental scars of war. And in an unexpected way, VR is bringing the humanity back into healthcare. I will use the term "VR" throughout this book as shorthand for all of this. But when I use that term, understand that I am referring to the revolutionary new science of immersive therapeutics, not a headset. Calling it VR is just short and sweet.[*]

VR is revolutionary because it compels us to think of patients differently than we doctors typically do. Doctors tend to think about patients as broken machines. VR rejects this notion and makes the case that in medicine, people's subjective lives matter. Jaron Lanier, the noted computer scientist who originally coined the term "virtual reality," says it best:

> VR is the most humanistic approach to information. It suggests an inner-centered conception of life, and of computing, that is almost the opposite of what has become familiar to most people, and that inversion has vast implications. . . . Most technology reinforces the feeling that reality is just a sea of gadgets; your brain and your phone and the cloud computing service all merging into one superbrain. . . . VR is the technology that instead highlights the existence of your subjective experience. It proves you are real.[1]

There's a lot to unpack in Lanier's vision of humanistic VR. This book will tell you something about what that quote means, from the perspective of a physician who has used VR for years alongside traditional

---

[*] A technical definition of VR is the use of a head-mounted display to interact with a computer-generated environment in a realistic manner. A related term is *augmented reality*, or AR, where virtual elements are superimposed over the real world (think of the popular game *Pokémon Go*, where cartoon characters appear to coexist with people). Some use the term *extended reality*, or XR, as an umbrella for VR/AR. Others prefer *spatial computing* as a broad term that describes blending immersive tech with the three-dimensional world. The US Food and Drug Administration now calls this field MXR, short for *medical extended reality*. For simplicity, I will call all of this VR. I will also intersperse the term *immersive therapeutics*, which means using VR for treatment purposes as opposed to education or simulation.

medical treatments. VR is not just for gamers anymore; it is a new type of medicine that not only has potential to heal but also can strengthen the bond between doctor and patient.

My own virtual leap revealed how VR can hijack the brain and create a sense of psychological *presence*. When VR scientists speak of presence, they mean that VR has a unique ability to convey a sense of just "being there," wherever *there* happens to be. It might be relaxing on a beach or soaring in a hang glider or swimming with dolphins or, in my case, tumbling off the side of a building. VR can even cause people to think and feel like another person altogether. In these pages, we'll see how VR enables people with depression to assume the body of Sigmund Freud and engage in self-counseling through his persona, allows patients with anorexia to experience life by way of a healthy avatar, and teleports people outside their own body so that they may gain new insights about the nature of dying. In all of these cases, if the VR is any good, the user feels transported to a new virtual environment and temporarily accepts it as reality. When used in the right way, at the right time, and with the right patient, these virtual journeys can change mind and body for the better.

It turns out that our brains are designed to live in one reality at a time. Hard as I tried while standing atop that building, my brain could not occupy two worlds at once. It could not contemplate the vivid reality of imminent death while simultaneously accepting the bland reality of standing in a conference room. I was shockingly unable to separate real from virtual. That's the power of presence and, in a nutshell, the power of VR. All of its revolutionary potential tumbles out of its ability to compel a person's brain and body to react to a different reality.

This book also traces a personal journey of scientific discovery. As a traditional Western-trained physician, I had doubts that VR could ever become part of my medical practice. At first, the technology seemed more like a nifty optical illusion than a meaningful therapeutic. I wasn't sure how a headset built for gaming and entertainment could truly improve health. The prospect of jumping off that building made it clear to me that VR creates unparalleled experiences that can support marketable products like immersive video games. I wondered about what else it could do. Could it help reduce suffering? Could it ease anxiety or stress? If so, could it reduce physical and emotional pain? Could it help battle unchecked narcotic abuse? I thought about the technology itself, which today is portable and relatively cheap. Could it extend care to people who do not have access to a clinic or therapist? By supplementing or replacing drugs, could VR somehow reimagine the boundaries of traditional Western medicine? What would healthcare look like if we took VR seriously?

For decades, a small cadre of scientists at elite universities have been quietly answering these questions. These pioneers, like Walter Greenleaf at Stanford and scores of others profiled in this book, have discovered the surprising health benefits of VR for ailments ranging from burn injuries to stroke to PTSD to schizophrenia to existential anxiety at the end of life, and more. Over five thousand studies reveal that VR has an uncanny ability to diminish pain, steady nerves, and boost mental health—all without drugs and their unwanted side effects.

Until recently, the technology has been too expensive, unreliable, and unwieldy for the research to translate beyond the pages of academic journals and doctoral dissertations. Now that's all changed. In the past five years, multinational companies such as Facebook, Google, HP, HTC Vive, Sony, and Samsung have invested billions of dollars into developing and expanding the VR industry. As a result, explosive advances have been made in delivering low-cost, portable, and high-quality VR to the masses. Goldman Sachs projects that VR will generate $80 billion in revenue by 2025.[2] We have reached an inflection point where the technology is cheap enough, its quality good enough, and the science voluminous enough to think seriously about leveraging VR to improve human health at scale.

My lab at Cedars-Sinai Medical Center in Los Angeles, and others like it, has been on a journey to study whether and how VR can improve health. In the process of doing so, we created one of the largest medical VR programs in the world. After treating several thousand patients, our team has learned a lot about whether, how, and when to use this technology to support clinical outcomes. By observing how VR influences cognition, we are learning new and surprising ways to optimize health choices, reduce medications, and train more empathic doctors. I wrote this book to describe these findings to a larger audience. I also wrote this book to give voice to patients benefiting from VR and to tell their stories. My hope is to advance this new field of medicine while acknowledging the decades of research and development that laid the foundations for translating VR science into this new clinical reality.

In these pages, I will reveal how we are using VR in the emergency department to help patients with panic attacks, treating women in labor who are seeking to avoid an epidural, and managing patients with orthopedic injuries. I discuss how VR can alleviate the worst kind of pain. I describe how VR can help treat irritable bowel syndrome, support stroke rehabilitation, assist patients undergoing dental procedures, steady tremors, and engage patients with dementia. I tell the story of how we teamed up with a local church to help parishioners lose weight, avoid salt, and lower blood pressure.

But VR also has risks. I have used VR to treat panic attacks, and have also inadvertently *caused* them with VR. I have seen people become dizzy and nauseous while flying over virtual landscapes. I've seen VR rekindle dark memories in victims of abuse. It can confuse children and the elderly. It can disorient people or cause them to fall. And then there's the more pernicious risk of overpromising and under delivering. I've heard Silicon Valley promoters hail the curative power of VR for all manner of disease. But VR has its limits and we must acknowledge them, understand the evidence supporting VR, and remain optimistic yet cautious about how best to harness this new digiceutical.[3] VR can't always cure what ails you. We can't just VR-away disease. But when used wisely, VR can supplement our ability to heal and help make life worth living.

In the process of telling these stories, *VRx* summarizes hundreds of studies, including our own published work, into actionable insights. The book reviews the evidence supporting therapeutic VR and provides judicious instruction on how to use this immersive technology as a complement to traditional medicine while minimizing risks.

Along the way, we will examine how VR affects the inner workings of the mind, explore the bounds of modern neuroscience, confront the bioethics and risks of VR, recognize the limits of using this technology for patient care, consider how to regulate the burgeoning "VR pharmacy" of immersive digital therapeutics, and predict how VR could impact the practice of medicine for years to come.

I am a physician with expertise in clinical medicine, digital health science, public health, and health economics. But I am not a computer scientist, electrical engineer, or clinical psychologist. This book is about patients and healthcare; it's about whether, when, and how to integrate VR within the very human experience of being sick; it's about how to make doctors more effective and patients better informed when using immersive therapeutics. My goal in this book is to explore the intersection between medicine and VR and to assess the current impact and future potential of this evolving clinical science from my perspective as a doctor. The reader seeking deeper expertise about the theory, history, and computer science of VR is encouraged to review the references included at the back of this book.

At its core, VR is a tool that modifies perception. When used to correct perceptions that undermine health, VR becomes a radical new therapy to help alleviate suffering from the most intractable diseases of mind and body. In Part I: Our Bodies, Our Selves, we explore the science of VR and discuss how this immersive technology is challenging neuroscientists, psychologists, and philosophers to rethink what it means to be a conscious self. The traditional view of consciousness is that it resides only in the brain. But modern neuroscience reveals the body is more than a mere support scaffolding for the brain; it is the extracranial foundation of our thinking mind. We need our bodies to have our minds. This theory, called embodied cognition, offers a framework to explain how VR alters mind, body, and consciousness through four therapeutic mechanisms that we will consider in Part I. Understanding these mechanisms not only reveals how the brain and body work in tandem, but it also justifies why Western medicine should expand to include VR as a legitimate, science-based intervention for afflictions like anxiety, depression, chronic pain, fibromyalgia, obesity, schizophrenia, and dementia, among many other common disorders.

Next, Part II: Virtual Medicine illustrates how the science of immersive therapeutics is being put to use in clinical practice. We travel to Cedars-Sinai Medical Center, my home base, to learn how VR is allowing our patients to escape the hospital and benefit from positive and emotionally enriching experiences. Through these stories, I describe our lessons learned using VR as a mind-body portal to reduce physical and mental distress. We'll then consider how best to personalize VR in a way that is safe and effective. If VR is truly a new therapy, then it is time to develop and regulate a VR pharmacy. I explain how our team and others are developing virtual pharmacies to tailor immersive therapeutics to individual patients.

Part III: Brave New World explores the humanistic implications of medical VR, highlights new opportunities for training doctors to more effectively deliver care with VR, and envisions how virtual medicine could change our daily life for years to come. I believe that VR has potential to strengthen the humanity in healthcare. It enables doctors to regard patients *as people*; it forces us to rethink the role of doctors as mind-body healers. At first blush, that might seem like an unlikely thesis. In a world of big data analytics, artificial intelligence, and algorithmic diagnostics, medicine is beginning to feel decidedly unhuman. But VR is a technology unlike any other. In Part III, we explore why VR is an *empathy machine* that allows doctors to engage more meaningfully with their patients and allows patients to become more empathic with themselves.[4]

VRx concludes by exploring the frontiers of therapeutic VR and forecasting how this new field could influence the practice of medicine for years to come. The capacity of VR to engage the embodied mind will only expand in the future. VR will help people using opioids to lower their doses by wearing a sensor that signals the mind when narcotics are paralyzing the gut. Paraplegics will relearn to walk with the help of VR-controlled exoskeletons. People suffering with anxiety or depression will use headsets equipped with artificial intelligence that senses mood and counters harmful emotions with precisely timed, contextually relevant immersive treatments. All of these technologies exist now. It's time to enter this world of virtual medicine.

One last thing: I didn't finish my story about scaling that virtual building. Did I ever jump? Well, sort of. I had to cheat. The VR headset was slightly ill-fitting, which afforded a sliver of light to enter beside my nose. I focused all my attention on the light and located a tiny patch of beige carpet on the floor—a stable point of reality in an otherwise dynamic virtual landscape. This was enough to break the illusion temporarily and permit me to take a shuffling baby step off the rig. And then I plummeted to my virtual death.[*]

---

[*] And it was all caught on video. You can watch the freefall here: www.virtualmedicine .org/freefall.

PART I

Our Bodies, Our Selves

As technology changes everything, we here have a chance to discover that by pushing tech as far as possible we can rediscover something in ourselves that transcends technology.

—Jaron Lanier, computer scientist, author, and the "father of VR," Microsoft Research

CHAPTER ONE

The Second Time I Died

I AM WEARING A CATSUIT WHILE RECLINING IN A CHAIR WITH MY LEGS kicked up on a coffee table in the research laboratory of Mel Slater, a professor of virtual reality at the University of Barcelona. Motion detectors and tiny vibration motors are affixed to my arms and legs. I am being tracked by an array of twelve cameras surrounding my chair that will soon inform a computer how my body is moving in space and time. Slater is standing behind me. A slight, bespectacled man straight out of central casting as the archetypal university professor, Slater speaks in a calm and light British accent. He is reviewing my final flight instructions for what is sure to be a most unusual journey. I've traveled six thousand miles from my home in Los Angeles for this moment.

"Just relax into the experience."

I trust him. I'm ready.

Slater's postdoc, Ramon Oliva, hands me a headset. I put it on and find myself in a comfortable living room with a lit fireplace, plush seats, and wood trimming. There is a mirror on the wall in front of me that reflects the image of my pixelated doppelgänger. And there's the coffee table under my feet, just where I left it.

"Okay, move your legs around on the table," says Oliva.

I oblige. In perfect synchrony, I see my own legs dance about on the digital tabletop. For a moment, I cannot tell whether those legs are mine. They *look* like my legs. They *act* like my legs. But *are they* my legs? I wiggle them back and forth. They move as expected. Yes, those are my legs. At least, I'm pretty sure they're my legs. If not, then whose legs could they be?

Next, little blue balls drop from the ceiling. Pop! I feel a ball hit my foot. A vibration engine in the suit fires at the same moment the virtual ball strikes my virtual body. Pop! Pop! Two more balls hit my left and right hand. Pop! Pop! Pop! Balls keep falling from the ceiling and tapping my limbs.

I think for a second: What is happening here? A computer somewhere in this room is running thousands of lines of code that are creating an illusion of spherical balls. Yet, those virtual balls—those pixelated clusters—are hitting my body with a very real physical force. I am *feeling* those digital balls. Those balls are real. This body is real. It is *my* body. The physical and virtual worlds are becoming indistinguishable. They are starting to feel like one unified existence.

I am now locked into my digital self. I have assumed what Slater calls full body ownership. The synchronous visual and tactile stimulation has convinced my brain that it now resides in a virtual head, in a virtual body, in a virtual room. My virtual feet are on a virtual coffee table. I see my body in a virtual mirror. I exist in this virtual world. This virtual world is a real world.

I will not soon forget what happens next. It is indelible, even mystical. I will do my best to describe it.

I start to move. And I mean *I* start to move, but my body stays put. In a steady backward flow, my personhood—my thinking self—begins to pull away from my body. I imagine sinews stretching, pulling, and snapping as my body resists the separation. It cannot hold on. I vacate my body and watch it as my consciousness drifts up toward the ceiling. I sense a brief existential crisis, a sort of Cartesian fit where my mind and body seek to reconcile the separation. For the first time in my life, I am disconnected from myself. I cannot tell if this is a physical or metaphysical cleavage, but it doesn't really matter. It *feels* as if I have been extracted from my body. I am floating like a balloon. Now I am up in the ceiling looking down upon my lifeless self. I am moving my hands, and those balls keep following me up to the ceiling and continue to strike my limbs. I've become an ethereal and disembodied entity hovering above my shell of a body below. That body down there is not moving. My arms are moving—I can feel them—but that body is not. I am in motion but that body is still. That body is unresponsive.

I am dead.

I am strangely entranced—even invigorated—by my virtual passing. I feel free from my body. And most confusing of all, I am no longer sure who the *I* is that's observing this phenomenal scene.

Where do you end and the world begin? Where is the frontier between self and other? Are we defined by corporeal boundaries? Or do we extend beyond the physical? And how can answering these questions help explain my out-of-body experience? Just what happened in my brain, and why? After literally rising from the dead, I needed some answers.

Generations of philosophers, cognitive psychologists, and neuroscientists have grappled with these questions about the nature of self. As an undergraduate I was fortunate to study Philosophy of Mind at Tufts University under the tutelage of Daniel Dennett, a renowned cognitive scientist and philosopher who was among the first to align diverse fields into a unified theory of consciousness. Dennett's work combines philosophy, psychology, and neuroscience to argue that what we experience as the mind is an emergent property of neurons oscillating in the brain. He says a lot more than that, but ultimately Dennett contends that physical phenomena and neurologic scintilla generate what we experience to be our conscious self. He argues that material stuff is the basis of all sensations, emotions, and cognitions. In other words, we end where our body ends, and the self emerges from the fantastic complexity of our wet inner world. Dennett's materialist argument, which is now shared by most modern neuroscientists, offers a framework for understanding my own out-of-body experience.[1]

Professor Dennett introduced me to the classic "brain-in-a-vat" thought experiment made famous in 1981 by Hilary Putnam,[2] an American philosopher who, like Dennett, spent much of his career studying the nature of mind. Putnam posed a curious question: How can you know that you're not just a disembodied brain floating in a vat of nutrients, wired up and connected to a computer that pumps your noggin full of artificial illusions simulating reality? He imagined a mad scientist who created a supercomputer that commandeers the brain into experiencing the phenomena of life. The result would be sensing the world as if you were a walking, talking entity, but, in fact, you would just be a brain floating in a vat. Putnam's thought experiment became the premise of *The Matrix* movie series, where people live in pods that nourish the body while the brain is occupied by a virtual reality supplied by sentient evil machines. In this dystopian world, the experience of life is just the result of electrical illusions.

What is often lost in discussing the brain-in-a-vat concept is that Putnam used his thought experiment to *disprove* that we are, in fact, brains in vats. His epistemic arguments are beyond the scope of this discussion, but suffice it to say, Putnam's thought experiment allows us to both contemplate the notion of computers simulating reality and to ponder what that means about the nature of self and how our brains operate. What was a mere thought experiment in 1981 is now something close to reality with advances in VR technology.[3]

Just consider my virtual out-of-body experience. Rather than Putnam's mad scientist in a lab, there was Professor Slater (who is certainly not mad) in his lab. Rather than some brain floating in a vat of chemicals connected to a computer, there was, well, *my* brain connected to a computer through sophisticated sensory feedback loops. Rather than lines of code convincing a floating brain that it is experiencing a spiritual event, there were lines of code convincing *my* brain that it was experiencing a spiritual event. The brain-in-a-vat is no longer a thought experiment; it is a real neurophysical experiment. And thinking about it can tell us something profound about the slippery relationship between what we see and what we feel.

So just what happened in my brain? How did a set of motion sensors, a bank of cameras, a VR headset, and a computer cause my brain to experience an ego-dissolving, selfhood-busting, mystical event that left me both dead and alive while spread apart in a virtual living room? How did I end up in *The Matrix* ?

The answer has something to do with that mirror in Professor Slater's virtual living room. At first, I saw a reflection that made sense. I moved my body in space, and the reflection responded in kind, abiding the familiar laws of motion I've experienced my whole life. But then, like a magic trick, my reflection in that same mirror no longer made sense. I saw an inanimate body in that mirror. I watched myself pass through my motionless avatar and float behind it. I watched myself die. In the process, Slater's brain-in-a-vat computer simulation coaxed my brain into accepting an alternative reality. I was no longer able to tell where my body ended and the world began. My physical sense of self in the world—my literal coordinates in space—were temporarily unbounded, allowing my mind freedom to roam in ways it never knew were possible. Even now, long after the demonstration finished, I feel differently about my relationship to my body. I can now say I've felt an out-of-body experience, and I can testify that it reduced my own personal fear of death, if even just a tiny bit. Understanding *how* it did this offers insights into the power of VR to alter mind and body, in both the short and long term. It helps us explain the unique ways that immersive therapeutics can improve health.

We begin this scientific journey by contemplating how a dime-store mirror can profoundly transform human consciousness.

The discovery that culminated in my mystical experience in Barcelona traces back to an astonishing yet simple study conducted by V. S. Ramachandran in the mid-1990s at the University of California, San Diego.[4] A clinical neurologist and cognitive neuroscientist, Ramachandran was struggling to find an effective treatment for his patients suffering from phantom limb pain. Phantom limb is a maddening condition where people who suffer an amputated arm or leg continue to feel its ghostly presence long after the appendage is gone. For some patients, the phantom limb feels extremely painful—even spastic—like a hand balled up in a tight fist. Yet, there is no hand. There is no fist. In a bid to restore a sense of corporeal wholeness, the brain hallucinates the continued presence of a false limb.

Ramachandran and his colleagues had a conceptual breakthrough: if they could just fool the brain into thinking there was a *real* limb present after all, then they could offer patients a chance to regain control over their phantom sensations. The researchers did this by creating a simple and elegant device they called a virtual reality box, also dubbed a mirror box. In the case of a missing arm, it worked like this: patients placed their remaining, healthy arm through a hole cut in the side of a cardboard box. The box was split into two chambers with a mirror affixed vertically along the separation wall. When positioned correctly, the healthy hand reflected off the mirror and created the appearance of a complementary second hand exactly where it should be. The following image shows a healthy left hand reflecting off the mirror and simulating the presence of a healthy right hand. If you look carefully, you can see that the right arm does not extend into the box at all; the amputated stump stops short of the box, yet the reflected hand appears like an extension of the missing limb.

Ramachandran's first mirror box patient was a fifty-five-year-old man with unrelenting sensations of spasms in his phantom arm. These sensations persisted for months after the amputation. The patient viewed his illusory hand in the mirror while attempting to resurrect his phantom hand. On the very first attempt, he reported that all movement had come back into his missing limb and that the pain subsided. Soon after, Ramachandran tested the mirror box with a twenty-eight-year-old man also suffering from severe phantom limb pain. His pain had persisted for nine years after a traumatic arm amputation. The first time he tried the box, the patient described the experience as "mind boggling"

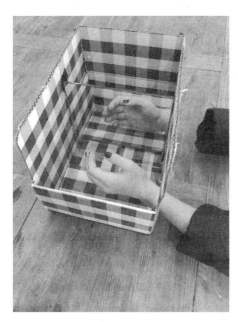

Ramachandran's "virtual reality box."

and reported that his arm was "plugged in again" and no longer felt "like it's lying lifeless in a sling."[5] After three weeks of therapy, his phantom arm pain disappeared completely. It never returned. And with that single experiment, Ramachandran laid the scientific groundwork for therapeutic VR. He had discovered a rudimentary yet revolutionary technique to alter consciousness.

Much of the promise of VR is predicated on the fundamental insights gained by the mirror box experiments. Our sense of self—our perception of where we physically begin and end—is a substrate for feelings like pain and anguish, and it can be easily manipulated. Our very coordinates in space, which we take for granted as objective, essential, and absolute, are less certain than we might imagine. Virtual experiences have a remarkable ability to undermine certainty. This power may confuse or deceive, but if employed properly, it can strengthen cognitions and enhance well-being.

Admittedly, it seems like a big jump between using a mirror for a phantom limb and teleporting an entire body to the ceiling. To tell the next part of this story, we turn to the unlikely combination of a rubber hand, two paintbrushes, and a knife.

When Henrik Ehrsson was a child he wondered whether God had played a trick on him by placing his soul in his brother's body, and vice versa. He felt there had been a cosmic mix-up that left his mind in the shell of the wrong person. This curious thought caused Ehrsson to ask some heady questions as a child, like, "How do I know that this is my body, and not my brother's body? Why does it feel like I am located inside this body? And how do I experience the world through my own eyes?"[6]

So this little boy became interested in the brain and what it means to have a conscious human mind. He wondered how we can recognize that our limbs are part of our own body, and how we sense the physical location of our self within our body, and not elsewhere. Forty years later, Ehrsson is an esteemed professor of cognitive neuroscience at the Karolinska Institute in Sweden, where his lab is investigating the nature and boundaries of personhood. His provocative research challenges what it means to be a thinking mind within a physical body. Ehrsson's work is important because it provides the missing link between Ramachandran's mirror box and Slater's virtual out-of-body experience.

When Ehrsson began planning experiments to address his childhood curiosities, he came across a fascinating 1998 study published in *Nature* by Matthew Botvinick from the University of Pittsburgh and Jonathan Cohen from Carnegie Mellon University.[7] Inspired by the work of V. S. Ramachandran, Botvinick, and Cohen created a cognitive parlor trick that had the opposite effect of the mirror box illusion. Rather than disowning a false limb and extinguishing its misleading sensations, their experiment *induced ownership* of a false limb and removed ownership of a real limb. The bizarre result was a convincing illusion of transferring body ownership from one's real arm to a fake arm.

Here's how it worked: Botvinick and Cohen sat people down in a chair and asked them to rest their arms on a table. Then they positioned a vertical barrier between the subject's eyes and one arm, putting the limb out of sight. Next, they placed a lifelike rubber hand on the table near the real hand, but on the visible side of the vertical barrier. The subject could not see the real hand, but instead viewed a life-sized fake hand in nearly the same location as the true hand. Once the setup was complete, the

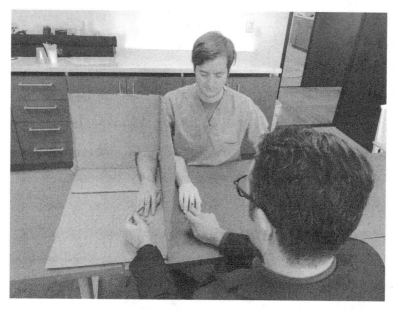

Experimental setup for the "rubber hand illusion."

researchers stroked the rubber hand and real hand at the same time using a pair of fine-tipped paintbrushes, taking care to synchronize the brush strokes as closely as possible. This photo shows the experimental setup.

Botvinick and Cohen found that before long, their research subjects were convinced the rubber hand was their own. They had embodied a gag appendage as an extension of the real body. When subjects were asked to close their eyes and point to their real hand, they were more likely to point to the fake hand, not their own, demonstrating the limb transfer illusion was complete. Just like with Ramachandran's work, the brain had been duped again, but this time into owning rather than disowning a false limb.

Ehrsson suspected this research could help satisfy his childhood questions. He set about studying just *how* the rubber hand illusion occurs and what it means about our sense of self. To achieve this, he placed research subjects into a functional magnetic resonance imaging (fMRI) scanner to take pictures of their brain during the rubber hand experiment.[8] The fMRI revealed that brain patterns shifted abruptly once the subject accepted ownership of the rubber hand. There were upticks in areas that involve integration of touch, vision, and movement. Activity in an area called the premotor cortex most closely reflected the feeling of hand ownership. After a lifelong pursuit of his childhood curiosities, Ehrsson discovered a place in the brain where we feel the sense of physical embodiment.

And then came the knife part. In another dramatic experiment, Ehrsson used the same rubber hand procedure as before, but this time he pulled out a knife and threatened to injure the fake hand. Not surprisingly, people freaked out.[9] The rubber hand illusion is so authentic that research subjects jump back, their heart rate speeds up, and they begin to sweat. On fMRI scanning, the pain-anticipation areas of the brain light up, demonstrating an immediate, hardwired response to the perception of impending bodily harm. Nobody was actually in danger in these experiments, but their brains weren't taking any chances.

Ehrsson didn't stop there. He asked an intriguing question: If we can fool the brain into owning or disowning a false hand, then why can't we trick it into accepting an *entire false body*? Can we literally body swap using the modern equivalent of smoke and mirrors? And what is that modern equivalent? Ehrsson had a candidate technology in mind: a VR headset.

There is something special about the first-person point of view. As I type these words, I see them through my eyes. Photons streaming off the words trigger cells in my retina to fire signals that reach the visual cortex in the back of my brain. My visual cortex interprets the neural fusillade as words on a computer screen. My brain assigns meaning to the words, checks for typos, ensures they are expressing what I am trying to say, and so forth. I only know this experience through my eyes and my body. My first-person vantage point is intrinsic to who I am. It is hard for me to imagine experiencing these words through someone else's eyes and body, just as it would be hard for you to imagine experiencing these words through my eyes and body.

What if we wanted to swap perspectives and experience the world through each other's eyes? How could we do it? We might each wear a first-person camera and livestream our view. I could watch a monitor and see what you are seeing, and vice versa. But I wouldn't really feel like I was in your head, or using your eyes, or occupying your body. Nor would you feel the same in reverse. We would both just see what the other person was seeing.

Henrik Ehrsson thought about these same questions and realized a VR headset might offer a solution. He devised another experiment where the research subject wore a head-mounted display and gazed straight ahead while sitting in a chair. There was a stereoscopic camera behind the chair that beamed livestream images to the headset. This arrangement allowed the seated individual to see an immersive view of his or her body from behind, as if experiencing the scene through the eyes of a third-person observer in close proximity. Next, Ehrsson tapped the chest of the research participant with a stick while synchronously poking under the camera with a matching stick. This picture shows the experimental setup.[10]

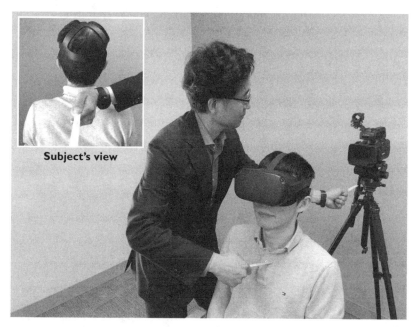

Subject's view

Experimental setup for the "phantom body illusion."

People in the chair felt displaced to the location of the camera behind their actual coordinates. They experienced a radical out-of-body illusion where they vacated their physical body. Rather than removing ownership of a phantom limb, as Ramachandran achieved with his mirror box, Ehrsson caused ownership over a *phantom body* using a souped-up version of the rubber hand illusion.

Ehrsson conducted additional experiments to explore the body-swap illusion. In one study, he used a VR headset to transport people into the body of a rubber mannequin.[11] Then he attacked the mannequin with a knife, causing people to react violently. In another experiment, he shrunk people down to the size of Barbie and Ken dolls, literally causing them to feel like Alice in Wonderland surrounded by oversized objects.[12] Other researchers followed suit, showing that people could feel a body swap with each other using a VR headset as the illusory conduit. An interdisciplinary group of scientists, artists, and designers created *The Machine to Be Another*, a program that allows anyone to experience the world from the viewpoint of another through a head-mounted display.[13] The program features a library of what the developers call embodied storytelling experiences. The effect is well captured by Aaron Souppouris, a reporter for *The Verge*, who described his experience of switching gender:

> I am no longer Aaron Souppouris. I am a woman. I am a stranger. I stare down at the mask I hold in my hands, struggling to comprehend how those hands, which are clearly not mine, are allowing me to feel its curves and cracks. As I glance at the mirror in front of me, my new lip piercing glimmers under the harsh fluorescent lights. This is not a fever dream, not a hallucination, not even a video game. This is *The Machine to Be Another*.[14]

After careful observation of these body-swap experiments, Ehrsson identified *three rules* that enable the illusion. First, he discovered that the tactile stimuli must be delivered simultaneously between the real and false bodies. If there is a delay between the visual and actual touches, then the illusion is violated. Second, the stimuli need to be in the same direction. For example, the brain will not accept a virtual hand if it's stroked in the opposite direction of the real hand. Third, the virtual body needs to be very near the real body. If there is too much distance between the bodies, then the brain sees through the ruse. He called these key principles the *temporal rule*, *spatial rule*, and *distance rule* of body transfer.[15] When these three conditions are met, the brain is tricked into relocation.

Ehrsson's three rules offer a fundamental recipe for shedding the self. When all three criteria are satisfied we can patch into a new reality. Now think back to my out-of-body experience. Professor Slater fooled my brain using a combination of insights from Ramachandran's mirror box, Botvinick and Cohen's rubber hand, and Ehrsson's body-swap rules. Using the temporal rule, he synchronized the virtual ball strikes with the sense of touch that was created by vibration engines in the catsuit. Using the spatial rule, he coordinated the directional movements of my actual and virtual legs on the coffee table. Using the distance rule, he started the illusion very close to my own body—even *inside* my own body—and only then distanced myself from, well, myself. The result was a complete out-of-body experience.

But more than that, Slater induced a transcendent, even mystical, experience. It was more than a parlor trick. Beyond the physical wonder of spatial displacement, I had the emotional experience of confronting mortality. Just how did one lead to the other? It is this leap, from sensorial to emotional, where we begin to appreciate not just the physical impact of VR on the body but also its therapeutic benefits on the mind.

Speaking of leaps, I have virtually died twice in this book so far: first, after virtually leaping off a building. Then, again, after teleporting to the ceiling and observing my lifeless body from above. I was petrified in the first instance. I felt oddly transcendent in the second. In both cases, VR created powerful cognitions *and* strong physical sensations. These were full body experiences.

I don't think I was a brain-in-a-vat in either scenario. That just can't be right. Both experiences required that I have a body, not just a brain. I reside in a physical body, and that body affects everything I think and know. It is shortsighted to think of the brain as a bundle of nerves riding atop a physiologic machine. Instead, it is an integrated part of the machine that is intertwined and harmonized within the body as a whole.

In 1641 the French philosopher René Descartes famously concluded, "I think, therefore I am." It was his way of saying that he believed the thinking mind was made of immaterial stuff that was categorically separate from the physical material of the body. Descartes proposed that the mind and body interfaced at the pineal gland, a tiny structure buried deep in the brain. This view became known as dualism, meaning the mind and body are two distinct entities. Cartesian dualism dominated Western theories of mind for centuries. Turns out it was wrong. Modern neuroscience suggests the story is more complex and interesting. Our sense of self—our very consciousness—depends not only on having a brain but also on having a body. We need our bones, tendons, ligaments, viscera, and sense organs to be conscious.

You know this to be true if you've been to a rock concert and *felt* the low-octave notes of a bass guitar pulsing through you. You can experience the same thing with the reverberating chords of a cathedral's pipe organ. We can "hear" these instruments with our body. The sounds seem like they come straight up from the floor and into your seat. Somehow, the physical experience of a vibrating derriere generates sound in our mind.

Not just sensations, but even judgments are modified by the physical state of our bodies. In a remarkable experiment conducted by University of Cambridge neuroscientist Simone Schnall, research subjects stood at the bottom of a steep hill and were instructed to rate its angle of ascent.[16] On its face, this task seems like a test of geometric reasoning more than a measure of bodily fitness. But Schnall had a theory that the amount of glucose circulating in the body might affect judgment about the steepness of the hill. After all, if you have more energy-producing glucose coursing through your veins, then you might be better prepared to size up and ascend the incline. The research team divided subjects into two groups: one received a purple drink full of glucose, and the other received a purple drink full of artificial sweetener. Sure enough, those receiving the sugar boost were more likely to rate the angle of the hill correctly. In contrast, the sugarless group rated the hill to be steeper than it actually was.

Even the bacteria in your colon can affect how you think and feel. As a gastroenterologist, I spend a lot of time studying the connections between the gastrointestinal system and the brain.[17] Both sides communicate all day long. On the gut side, billions of bacteria affect us in unexpected ways. My former colleague Kirsten Tillisch discovered that replacing bad bacteria in the gut with good bacteria can change how the brain responds to stress.[18] Compared to a group of research subjects who didn't consume a probiotic yogurt, those who did exhibited diminished activity in the brain's emotion centers when exposed to faces of people in distress. This suggests a dampened fear response. Such experiments demonstrate that the mind is very much dependent on the body, and in this case, on the meta-notion of bodies within the body.

All of these examples support a theory called embodied cognition, which is the idea that everything we think about and know is a result of not just having a brain but also because that brain is connected to the rest of the body.[19] MIT neuroscientist Alan Jasanoff describes this theory as "thinking, outside the box," meaning that our sense of consciousness begins well outside of our head.[20] The body is an extracranial extension of our brain that collects signals from the world around us and from within us, packages them up, and sends them to the central processing unit upstairs. This affects what we think about, what we know, and how we feel.

Although our brains are cooped up in solidified bunkers, they are tightly bound to the rest of our bodies through an extensive network of sense organs. We see, hear, smell, taste, and touch our way into consciousness. *We need our body to have our mind.* Whether it be through consuming glucose to sharpen analytic skills, using probiotics to dampen a fear response, or wearing a headset and vibration motors to trigger an out-of-body experience, we can modify our mind by modifying our body.

Think about how VR caused my pair of virtual deaths. The first time I died, VR changed my perceived coordinates to the top of a building where I grappled with the emotional fallout of an existential crisis. This mental impact caused a profound physical impact. My heart raced, my blood pressure rose, my skin moistened, and my jaw clenched. I had no way of controlling this automatous response. It just happened. Then my body sent a barrage of signals back up to my brain through a process called interoception, where a vast network of sensors alerts the brain when things seem off inside the body. The signals overwhelmed my brain and triggered a sense of fear. This led to embodied cognitions, like thinking I should keep my body still, step closer to the wall behind me, and steady my nerves. I quickly scribed a mental narrative of imminent death. My selfhood had been threatened by a plastic headset.

My second virtual death was different. In that case, the immersive experience engaged two senses—vision and touch—to generate a complex response that felt like a mix between placidity and nervousness. My breathing relaxed and I felt a sense of comfort, yet my heart rate increased and my pupils (most likely) dilated to capture the extraordinary scene. I don't have a picture of my face during the experiment, but I imagine it had a look of amazement. I would guess my blood pressure rose slightly—at least at first—to prepare for escape if things didn't go well. This physiologic response sent interoceptive signals to my brain that heightened awareness and created a sense of mysticism; that's the best word I can find to describe vacating my body. I am no mystic, but scholars of mysticism identify several shared attributes of all mystical experiences. They are ineffable, if not impossible, to express in common language; they feel as though the ego steps aside, leaving room for new cognitions to emerge that are normally suppressed under the domineering watch of a ruminating self; there is a sense of certainty that the perception is real and meaningful; and they generate feelings of joy and satisfaction.[21] My own out-of-body experience fulfilled all of these criteria. The feeling was neither religious for me nor demanding of a supernatural cause. But it sure *felt* that way. I could see how others might experience it as a spiritual event.

Somehow, the act of virtually dying left me with a new cognition about mortality. It prepared me, in a small but meaningful way, for when the real event inevitably occurs. Professor Slater managed to associate a traditionally negative sentiment—contemplating one's own death—with an unexpectedly transcendent experience, all by tweaking my body with a headset and vibration motors. Those simple physical nudges caused embodied cognitions that left me with a profound new insight: I learned that dying is not a purely negative event.

It could have been different, by the way. If Professor Slater had been an evil scientist, the sort imagined by Hilary Putnam in his original brain-in-the-vat thought experiment, I might now be terrified by death. The same transcendent simulation could have been horrifying. Instead of placidly teleporting into the sky, I could have plummeted into fire, or watched my body become decimated, or who knows what? Perish the thought. Thankfully, Slater dialed up a more beneficent use of VR. And that's the point: because VR is a tool that profoundly alters mind, body, and consciousness, it can be wielded to achieve vastly different effects.

In the case of my out-of-body experience, nothing about that simulation *proved* that death is not purely negative. VR did not teach me a scientific fact about the nature of dying. Instead, my new mind-set about death resulted from an association Slater created by virtue of how he constructed the scene: I died in a comfortable and quiet room, the process of leaving my body was serene, there was no drama or threatening music or pain, and the feeling of hovering over my body was ethereal. VR made me think death is not that scary because that's how Slater engineered the experience. This is a crucial point, because it goes to the notion that designing virtual worlds allows us to create specific associations and experiences that confront particular problems. In healthcare, where people can suffer from debilitating physical and mental symptoms, VR can recalibrate how those symptoms are perceived and, in some cases, address their root causes. We will consider examples of that idea throughout the book.

So, for me, Slater built a virtual world that taught me something profound and durable about the nature of death. Those five minutes in Barcelona were an unexpected gift. By paradoxically fearing death just a little bit less, I can enjoy life just a little bit more. In short, VR changed my mind.

It's not just me. In a pioneering study titled "A Virtual Out-of-Body Experience Reduces Fear of Death," Professor Slater performed a controlled trial comparing two types of extracorporeal events.[22] Subjects in the experimental group underwent a fully embodied death similar to what I described at the beginning of this chapter. Those in the control group also floated up to the ceiling like I did, but rather than looking down upon a lifeless body, they instead saw a *living* body that they could still control from afar.[*] Once the participants completed their assigned procedure, Slater assessed the degree of perceived body separation and measured the resulting fear of death. To avoid biased responses, the research participants had no idea prior to enrolling that they'd be asked about death anxiety. In case you were wondering, there is indeed an official "Fear of Death Scale." Here is the key question from the survey:

> What level of worry or anxiety do you have for the following aspects related to your own death?
> - The total isolation of death
> - The shortness of life
> - Missing out on so much after you die
> - Dying young
> - How it will feel to be dead
> - Never thinking or experiencing anything again
> - The disintegration of your body after you die

Slater discovered that subjects who abandoned a lifeless body reported a lower fear of death versus those who maintained control over their avatar. Slater even accounted for religiosity in his analysis. He found no relationship between religious convictions and fear of death resulting from the out-of-body experience. The cognitive effect was unrelated

---

[*] This video depicts the two conditions of the experiment: www.virtualmedicine.org /out-of-body.

to whether the subject was a theist or atheist, suggesting an a-religious phenomenon.

In an elaborate follow-up study published in 2018, Slater placed research subjects on a fantastical virtual island where they embodied alien life forms.[23] He grouped three strangers at a time to interact and cooperate in the virtual world. Meanwhile, in the real world, the participants sat in separate soundproof rooms and were disallowed from meeting in person. They explored the island and performed collaborative survival tasks over the course of six sessions during the weeklong experiment. Their alien bodies grew older throughout the study, beginning as children and progressing into advanced age in a simulated natural lifespan. Each participant witnessed the virtual death of their companions, and then experienced personal death at the end of the week. Similar to the earlier study, each participant detached from their body and viewed their motionless self from above. But this time, they also watched successive flashbacks that had been unwittingly recorded during their virtual life. Finally, the life review faded to black, a bright light emerged in its place, and the disembodied participants entered an illuminated tunnel that led to a final resting place. Having experienced this myself in Slater's lab, I can attest that it's a striking and compelling journey.

Slater repeated this experiment with multiple teams to build his experimental cohort. Then he compared life views among the VR participants versus a control group that did not experience the virtual island. The two groups completed an extensive questionnaire called the "Life Changes Inventory." It measured a range of beliefs about everything from reverence for life to acceptance of and empathy toward others to concerns with questions of social justice to interest in self-reflection. Slater found that people who experienced the cooperative virtual island expressed higher life-change scores than those in the control group. After living and dying in the immersive world, participants were more beneficent, self-accepting, and concerned about others. They also reported a higher sense of life purpose. Although the study was small, with only thirty-two participants, Slater offered evidence that VR can profoundly change minds for the better.

In this chapter, we have explored how VR alters what we think and feel. By simulating a first-person perspective and leveraging the power of virtual embodiment, VR modifies our experience of the world. It is a tool that can teach us about who we are and how our body and brain jointly support a conscious self.

The scientific discoveries described in this chapter set the stage for explaining how VR can improve health. VR is a technology that modifies perception. When used to recalibrate unhealthy perceptions, VR becomes a radical new therapy with potential to alleviate suffering from intractable diseases of mind and body. Throughout the rest of Part I, I will review four groups of diseases that VR can treat, each through one of four therapeutic mechanisms.

Chapter 2 addresses how VR is helping people with anxiety and depression through its ability to *promote cognitive flow*, the first of the four therapeutic mechanisms. Known colloquially as "being in the zone," cognitive flow is a feeling of being immersed, energized, and fully engaged in an activity that seems fluid and effortless. When people with anxiety or depression enter a flow state, they can disconnect from their inner critic and free their mind to operate without the constraints of self-judgment. Research shows that VR can help achieve flow by way of loosening a rigid mind in favor of a softened and freer conscious experience. If this sounds a bit like how LSD or magic mushrooms work, it's because VR shares a lot in common with psychedelics: both can create otherworldly, even mystical experiences, and both create multisensory illusions that stir the brain. VR is a hallucination machine with potential to free an overburdened mind. In Chapter 2, we will study examples where doctors and scientists are using this capability to treat phobias, lower anxiety, manage post-traumatic stress disorder, and combat depression.

Chapter 3 examines how VR *dampens inner pain signals*—its second therapeutic mechanism. We'll discover how VR directs the mind away from pain signals, nips pain in the bud at its source, and speeds up the perception of time for people suffering through pain episodes. Chapter 3 reviews the expanding evidence that VR can reduce pain for conditions like fibromyalgia, irritable bowel syndrome, and burn injuries.

Chapter 4 examines VR's third therapeutic mechanism, *strengthening self-identity*. This mechanism addresses two conditions marked by an eroded sense of self: schizophrenia and dementia. Rather than loosening a rigid mind, VR tightens a loose sense of self. Schizophrenia is considered to arise in part from an eroded identity; sufferers may lack a unified sense of self, feel as if they do not exist in the world, or perceive their inner dialogue to be public and available to others. Patients with dementia also suffer from a disorganized identity, albeit for different reasons. In both cases, VR is showing promise by strengthening self-identity, enabling more organized thinking, and helping patients to establish meaningful connections with the world around them.

There is also a group of conditions marked by a loose connection between mind and body where people struggle to recognize important internal signals. For example, obesity occurs in part when the mind overrides signals from the stomach that it is full. Research shows that anorexia nervosa has the opposite effect. For these conditions, VR works through its fourth therapeutic mechanism of *enhancing healthy body attention*. In Chapter 5, I will describe examples where VR is being used to manage eating disorders by fine-tuning perceptions of the body.

First up is the therapeutic mechanism for helping people with anxiety and depression. Let's consider why VR is like a digital psychedelic and examine what that means for treating a group of conditions that afflict nearly half of humankind.

CHAPTER TWO

The Self Blends

M Y MIND CHATTERS A LOT. IT CRITIQUES, FRETS, NAGS, AND OTHER-
wise distracts me from what I'm doing. Your mind probably
chatters, too. Neuroscientists call this our "default mode" of thinking.
Freudians call it the ego self. Zen Buddhists call it the monkey mind—
the part of your psyche that's always making a fuss, as if jabbering pri-
mates are leaping about from tree to tree in your head. Whatever you call
it, this part of your brain can be annoying. Worse still, when your inner
dialogue ruminates about potential threats, agonizes about relationships,
or worries about work deadlines, it can undermine your quality of life.
How we respond to and control our monkey mind determines, to a large
degree, how effective we are as people and how well (or unwell) we feel
physically, emotionally, and socially. This chapter is about how VR tames
the overthinking mind.

Amazing things happen when the monkey mind stops yammering.
Freed from the inner voice, the rest of the brain can relax, stretch out, and
explore in new and creative ways. Performance becomes effortless and
relaxed. Time slows down. Creativity blossoms as the brain makes new

connections. Scientists refer to this experience as a non-ordinary state of consciousness. You may know it as flow, a sense of just being "in the zone," as if the body and mind are operating so efficiently that they don't have time for self-reflection.

My near-death experience in Slater's lab was a non-ordinary state of consciousness. I described it as "mystical" in Chapter 1. Although I experienced a virtual death, the feeling was not tragic. Instead, it felt spiritual and invigorating. Time seemed to stand still. It felt good. I was in flow.

We've all had moments of flow. Sometimes they come when you're doing something challenging at work, or when you're connecting with someone in a fluid conversation. Comedians in flow can't help but be effortlessly hysterical. Scientists in flow see previously overlooked solutions to complex problems. Surgeons in flow operate as if their hands have a mind of their own.

I can recall many occasions when I entered flow while performing a medical procedure. On one occasion, I was working with a team of anesthesiologists and nurses to stop massive internal bleeding from a patient with a stomach ulcer. My job was to seal the ulcer from within by placing clips over the bleeding artery. The patient was extremely sick—so sick that we had to restart his heart in the middle of the procedure. This would have ordinarily been a very stressful situation. But we had entered a flow state, and everything slowed down. It felt like we had plenty of time to fix the problem. Technical maneuvers became easy and obvious. The clips fell precisely where they needed to fall. The team worked like an Indy pit crew. Everyone knew what to do, when to do it, and how to get it done. There were no egos in the room. There was no chattering, or second-guessing. Our monkey minds were dead. The patient lived.

Although flow is accessible to anyone, achieving flow is not so easy. If we could activate flow like turning on a spigot, then we'd all be in flow whenever we wanted and life would be amazing. Instead, most everyone is searching for how best to optimize their own personal flow state. Some people try to quiet their mind through meditation. Others through medication. Some try music therapy. Others use aromatherapy. Or acupuncture. Or yoga or hypnosis or . . . Pilates, cannabis, sweat lodging, deep tissue massage, orgasmic meditation, magnetic bracelets, rhythmic breathing, humor therapy, alcohol, extreme sports, talk therapy, video games, pornography, social media, TV bingeing, tobacco, gambling . . . and on, and on. Oh, and psychedelics, too. And of course, VR. More on those soon.

Taken together, these efforts at achieving flow comprise a $4 trillion "altered state economy."[1] Worldwide, we spend more money trying to quiet the monkey mind than we do on maternity care, humanitarianism aid, and K–12 education *combined*.[2] If flow were so easy to achieve, then it probably wouldn't be so expensive. But flow is elusive and there are barriers to entry like high cost, inadequate time, or difficulty finding the right state of mind.

Why do we spend so much time and money getting out of our collective head? The answer is twofold: flow has an addictive quality, as discovered by Mihaly Csikszentmihalyi, the renowned psychologist who originally coined the term "flow" in 1990.[3] But there's more to it than jonesing for another fix. We also seek flow to avoid the devastating consequences of its polar opposite—the ruminating mind. If flow is "the secret to happiness," as suggested by Csikszentmihalyi, then its opposite state is the root of anxiety, depression, and untold human anguish. The $4 trillion altered state economy is as much about avoiding misery as it is about seeking ecstasy. Authors Steven Kotler and Jamie Wheal aptly summarize the epidemic crisis of overthinking minds:

> Every issue we encounter, we try to solve by thinking. And we know it's not working. Even a quick glance at today's dire mental health statistics—the one in four Americans now on psychiatric medicines; the escalating rate of suicide for everyone from ages ten to seventy-eight—shows how critically overtaxed our mental processing is these days. We may have come to the end of our psychological tether. It might be time to rethink all that thinking.[4]

The overthinking mind can lead to mental anguish. For example, a patient with arachnophobia sees a spider and her brain kicks into hypervigilant overdrive. Or someone with depression interprets other people's actions and behaviors to mean he is a failure. In both cases, the ruminating mind spends too much time thinking and interpreting. It anguishes about possible future events (in the case of anxiety), or laments about past events (in the case of depression), but struggles to maintain focus on the moment. The thinking self "is not an unmitigated blessing," writes Duke University psychologist Mark Leary, author of *The Curse of the Self*. "It is single-handedly responsible for many, if not most of the problems that human beings face as individuals and as a species."[5]

Yet, at the same time, the thinking self is what defines us as human beings. "I think," said Descartes, "therefore I am." The same mental apparatus that triggers anxiety or depression also enables us to flourish as individuals and as a species. We don't want to shut down our self-reflective mind completely. Flow may feel great in short bursts, but if we were always in flow and unable to engage our self-reflective mind, we'd become ineffective stoners. We must strike a delicate balance here. When our thinking self is allowed to operate within its Goldilocks zone—that is, when it's not too hot, and not too cold, but just right—we become productive and high-functioning members of society. The goal, then, is to clear enough space for our mind to be productive, but also to erect guardrails that keep it from running out of control.

In this chapter, we explore how VR helps to keep our mind in balance. We discover how VR can promote a flow state that jailbreaks our mind when it's locked into unhealthy rumination. Then, once VR relieves us from mental gridlock, we can use it to reengage our mental apparatus in a more controlled and healthy manner. As we'll see, the result is a potent new therapy for anxiety and depression. But before we get there, we need to know why our minds become trapped in unhealthy cycles of rumination. Then we need to determine how to break free.

At this very moment, you are reading this book. This is the immediate now. Provided you're not distracted by something else, living in this moment briefly calms the angst of living outside the moment. This insight is nothing new—it forms the basis of all meditative traditions.

But few live by this advice. Instead, we frequently contemplate the future or the past, but less so the present. Our mind is often too busy planning, scheming, deciding, preparing, judging, and just *thinking* to appreciate the immediacy of now. Instead, moment-to-moment activities are governed by hardwired and largely unconscious behaviors. Just think about the last time you drove all the way home, pulled up to your parking space, and then wondered how in the world you got there. This phenomenon is so common it has a name: "highway hypnosis."[6] People are so distractible that each year nearly forty children die of vehicular heatstroke in the United States after being mistakenly left in a car by an otherwise caring parent.[7] It's hard to imagine a more devastating consequence of an absorbed mind.

Although it seems maladaptive to dwell on the past and future at the expense of the present, the self-reflective mind was not a curse back in the days when humans were hunter-gatherers. When our thinking mind first evolved forty thousand years ago, it bestowed humans with the ability to plan for the future, to make deliberate decisions, to be introspective, and to take the perspective of others. Those were incredible skills to have, particularly at a time when needs were limited to eating, reproducing, and perhaps a bit of socializing. Relationships were pretty simple. Our supercharged brain was more than equipped to handle life. But as life became more complex, particularly as humans evolved from hunter-gatherers living in the moment to farmers planning for the future, our mind had a lot more to worry about.

In their brilliant book, *The Distracted Mind*, neuroscientist Adam Gazzaley and psychologist Larry Rosen describe how our information-rich modern world can overwhelm our minds and diminish quality of life.[8] This occurs, they explain, through an ancient and inborn process called information foraging, where humans constantly seek out new information in the same way animals forage for food. According to this theory, when we encounter novel and interesting bits of data, our brains squirt out the same pleasure chemicals induced by eating tasty treats. These neurotransmitters, like dopamine and serotonin, reward our brain for mental wandering in the same way animals are rewarded for gathering food. It's as though our brain *enjoys* ruminating. If we run low on material to contemplate, then our instinct is to move on and find a richer knowledge pasture to support our information diet. For example, you might find yourself watching cable news, but after a while you get the gist and feel the need to turn the channel. And then turn it again. We constantly scour for fresh knowledge wherever we can get it, even if it means rapidly moving from one information source to another in order to keep our ruminating mind occupied.

Information foraging explains why it's so easy to lose track of the drive home. It explains why we are so distractible that we can't be happy with, say, a dinner conversation without feeling compelled to reach for a smartphone. We are surrounded by information sources, so we scurry about collecting and ingesting data to get the next hit of dopaminergic delight. But we often do so at the expense of focusing on the here and now. Gazzaley and Rosen conclude that we are "ancient brains in a high-tech world."[9]

Information foraging is controlled by the prefrontal cortex of the brain—the region right behind your forehead. The prefrontal cortex is a big part of what makes us uniquely human. It is the neural seat of executive functioning and cognitive control—a sort of "traffic controller" directing our attention and managing our decisions. As the last structure to evolve in the brain, the prefrontal cortex is the anatomical focus of the conscious self. Damage to this part of the brain leaves people unconcerned and detached from themselves and others. People with prefrontal injuries no longer self-reflect because there is no longer a self to reflect upon.

In 2001, a team of Washington University neurologists led by Marcus Raichle discovered that the prefrontal cortex is part of a larger brain network that controls the monkey mind.[10] They made this remarkable discovery while observing research subjects who were asked to lie down in an fMRI scanner and think about nothing at all. As one might imagine, most of the brain powered down when people cleared their mind. But unexpectedly, part of the prefrontal cortex perked up along with a group of deeper structures that control emotion and memory. Just as the research subjects were trying *not* to think, a unique brain network started thinking . . . a lot.

Raichle decided to call this group of brain structures the default mode network. This is a technical term that refers to the baseline buzzing that occurs when we're just trying to relax, yet the brain is busy foraging for new information and insights. Author Michael Pollan describes the default mode network as "the place where our minds go to wander—to daydream, ruminate, travel in time, reflect on ourselves, and worry."[11] When we are mindlessly driving home without paying attention, it's because the default mode network has drawn mental bandwidth from the rest of the brain, causing us to lose track of where we are and what we're doing. In essence, Raichle located the very source of our blabbering inner voice.

In a 2010 study conducted at Harvard University, psychologists Matthew Killingsworth and Daniel Gilbert found that the more time people spend in their default mode of thinking, the unhappier they become. "A wandering mind," they concluded, "is an unhappy mind."[12] If spending too much time in our head can make us miserable, then temporarily silencing the default mode network—the part that ruminates and worries—should lift our spirits. But we wouldn't want to shut it down forever. If we could at least *control* our default mode of thinking, by turning it on when helpful and turning it off when harmful, then we might achieve a better life balance.

Scientists determined that flow requires a state called transient hypofrontality, or temporary suppression of the prefrontal cortex.[13] With the prefrontal cortex off-line, the rest of the default mode network powers down, the self-critical mind quiets, and the brain is free to create new insights by connecting neural areas that normally do not communicate. Psychologists describe this as lateral thinking—a connect-the-dots form of cognition that bypasses the usual hub of consciousness dominated by the ego self. The result can be a profound sense of deep insight and transcendence.

But it's not easy to activate flow. Our usual way of thinking—our literal *default* way of thinking, as Raichle termed it—does not resemble anything like flow. We are accustomed to seeking out and interpreting data. So quieting this inner voice requires practice. Buddhist monks spend a lot of time in flow, but only because they accumulate well over forty thousand hours of meditative practice in their lifetime.[14] Professional athletes often describe being in flow, but they've spent decades honing their mind and body to perform without requiring a lot of conscious effort, if any. Same thing with concert pianists, or NASA astronauts, or heart surgeons. Whether it's in the performing arts, sports, or any other walk of life, it takes a lot of thought to be able to think without thinking.

Alternatively, some people take a shortcut to flow by taking risks. They might parachute out of an airplane or bungee jump or climb into a giant plastic orb and roll down a hill (yes, this is actually a thing; it's called zorbing). These intense and potentially dangerous activities overwhelm the self-reflective mind through brute force. The brain doesn't have a lot of time to ponder stuff when it's trying to survive. There is so much stimulation, in so little time, that the experience hijacks the foraging instinct with an information-rich distraction. There is no mental bandwidth left to consider anything outside the immediate experience, and certainly no time to ruminate about anything hypothetical or nonessential.

This is where VR steps in. VR requires no experience. There are no VR training classes. You just put on a low-cost headset and go. Yet, despite its simplicity and accessibility, VR can simulate rich experiences that would otherwise require years of practice, like deep meditation, or activities that are high risk, like jumping off a building. It's the immersive *presence* of VR—that embodied feeling of just "being there" and interacting with a new world—that entrains attention like no other audiovisual medium. Like zorbing, VR can overwhelm with novelty, but without the survival risk. Also, by covering the eyes and obscuring outside distractions, VR can more easily capture and hold attention because it completely controls the visual environment. These features confer a unique capability to achieve flow.

This explains why my virtual out-of-body experience in Mel Slater's lab felt mystical. Although I wasn't in a brain scanner at the time, here's what I think happened: first, the VR headset covered my face and removed external distractions. There was nothing competing for attention outside the immediate virtual environment. Next, the VR headset triggered my foraging instinct with an information-rich experience. This caused my prefrontal cortex to drop what it was doing and focus attention on the virtual environment. My brain redirected its power supply to support visual processing, leaving the prefrontal cortex with less energy to operate. The default mode network powered down. A sense of selflessness emerged. I lost track of time. My brain released norepinephrine—a natural stimulant—which amped my cardiovascular system and sharpened my focus. At the same time, my brainwaves—those oscillating electrical patterns in the brain that affect levels of consciousness—likely slowed from *beta wave* characteristics of agitated rumination to more relaxed *alpha waves*. As my brain rode the alpha waves into effortless flow, it released more dopamine, furthering the sense of pleasure. Next, my brain sunk deeper until it generated *theta waves*, which are usually reserved for REM sleep. The curious result was a sense of dreaming with my eyes wide open. Finally, my brain released its last batch of pleasure chemicals—oxytocin and serotonin—which produced an aura of tranquility. The net result was STER, an acronym coined by Kotler and Wheal that captures the four attributes of flow: selflessness, timelessness, effortlessness, and richness.[15] VR did this all within minutes. It required no preparation or practice on my part. I brought no special skills to Slater's lab. And despite dying in his virtual world, my passing was risk-free and safe. After all, I'm still here to write about it.

The ability of VR to promote cognitive flow mimics the effects of meditation and psychedelics, two very different modalities that affect the brain in similar ways. It's worth spending a moment to review how meditation and psychedelics work because it informs us about how VR treats anxiety and depression.

There are now hundreds of studies demonstrating that meditation alleviates a wide range of mental health conditions through its ability to induce flow. For the past decade, NYU neuroscientist Zoran Josipovic has been subjecting Buddhist monks to fMRI scans to examine what happens in their brains during meditation. He's shown that these super-meditators switch off their default mode network on a moment's notice, and then they keep it off for as long as they want.[16] Several other studies reveal the same thing: the more tranquil and selfless someone feels during meditation, the more likely that person is to have quieted the default mode network. Meditation is accessible to anyone, anywhere. But despite evidence that meditation does not require a monkish commitment to be helpful, many people are hesitant to begin a meditation practice or have trouble sticking with the program. Regardless, most people never come close to accumulating the years of practice achieved by Buddhist monks in Josipovic's fMRI studies.

Psychedelics also quiet the default mode network, albeit pharmacologically. Since the serendipitous discovery of LSD by a Swiss chemist working for Sandoz Laboratories in 1938, psychedelics have been recognized as flow-inducing compounds.[17] Hallucinogens like LSD and its close analogue, psilocybin (the active ingredient in so-called magic mushrooms), promote what users describe as nondual consciousness, meaning a sense of oneness between self and other. People who trip on psychedelics feel as if their body merges seamlessly with the outside world. Users might transform into a tree, or embody a piece of music, or become a color, or metamorphose into an animal. The self blends into otherness. The experience of losing oneself can be pleasurable, but not always— psychedelics can also cause "bad trips."

In his book, *How to Change Your Mind*, Michael Pollan chronicles the science of psychedelics and describes how these powerful hallucinogens can create life-changing experiences. Pollan took several of his own ego-dissolving trips to inform the book. His bizarre psilocybin experience offers a striking example:

> I watched as that familiar self began to fall apart before my eyes, gradually at first and then all at once. "I" now turned into a sheaf of little paper, no bigger than Post-its, and they were being scattered to the wind. But the "I" taking in this seeming catastrophe had no desire to chase after the slips and pile my old self back together. No desires of any

kind, in fact. Whoever I now was was fine with whatever happened. *No more ego?* That was okay, in fact the most natural thing in the world. And then I looked and saw myself out there again, but this time spread over the landscape like paint, or butter, thinly coating a wide expanse of the world with a substance I recognized as me.[18]

As I read this description of Pollan's amazing trip, I am reminded of my own out-of-body experience in Professor Slater's laboratory. In both cases a transcendent, virtual world replaced the real world. Both times the egocentric self was exchanged for a more distributed form of consciousness. Both challenged our understanding of physics, causing us to rethink our very coordinates in space and time. And despite the "seeming catastrophe" of losing our identities—however temporarily—we were both okay with it. Whereas Pollan arrived at his mystical state via pharmacology, I arrived via technology. But the phenomena of both trips bear a strong resemblance.

Just like with meditation, brain imaging confirms that psychedelics suppress the default mode network.[19] And once again, temporarily inhibiting the monkey mind pays dividends for health and well-being. Research shows that even a single dose of a psychedelic can help manage treatment-resistant depression, calm anxiety, break alcohol and smoking addiction, and treat obsessive compulsive disorder. The benefits are not only immediate, but appear to last for weeks, months, or in some cases years. For example, one study from Johns Hopkins University found that 80 percent of smokers quit after taking psilocybin, and more than two-thirds remained abstinent a year later—*after a single dose.*[20] Similarly, in another remarkable study conducted at Hopkins, neuroscientist Roland Griffiths used psilocybin to treat existential anxiety and depression among patients with life-threatening cancer.[21] He found that four out of five patients experienced meaningful improvements. Moreover, the effect was durable six months after one dose, suggesting a prolonged impact well beyond the immediate treatment period. In another study with healthy subjects, titled "Psilocybin Can Occasion Mystical-Type Experiences Having Substantial and Sustained Personal Meaning and Spiritual

Significance," Griffiths showed that one dose of the mind-altering hallu-cinogen changed people's life views for months after the treatment.[22] The results of his controlled experiment parallel Mel Slater's study, described in Chapter 1, where ego dissolution from VR induced a higher sense of life purpose, self-acceptance, and beneficence.

This raises some questions: Is VR a digital psychedelic? Can it de-liver the same ego-battling benefits as hallucinogens? If so, then perhaps VR could become a new mental health treatment with fewer barriers to entry. After all, psychedelics are currently only available through research studies or illicit recreational use; they are not yet FDA-approved. If VR could deliver pharmacology-free trips on par with psychedelics, then it could offer another "off button" for people who suffer from a ruminating mind. One way to find out would be to test VR against psychedelics and see what happens.

Anil Seth has done that study. A professor of neuroscience at the University of Sussex in the United Kingdom, Seth is among a small group of top scientists exploring the role of VR as a tool for manipulating and studying human perception. In 2017, Seth and his colleagues published an innovative trial pitting VR against psilocybin.[23] They used a computer software program developed by Google, called DeepDream, that radi-cally alters visual perceptions. Seth installed the software on a VR head-set to simulate the experience of tripping on psychedelics, but without the pharmacology. Volunteers in the study found themselves standing in the middle of the University of Sussex campus watching a bustling academic quad through the VR headset. The result was bizarre. The heads of pass-ersby were replaced by barking dogs, arms became ornate brass bells, tor-sos morphed into colorful parakeets, and walkways bore a shimmering purple surface straight out of a Dalí painting.[24] The researchers called their contraption the Hallucination Machine.

Seth compared the subjective experience evoked by VR to the ex-perience of a second group on psilocybin. Participants in both groups completed the "Altered States of Consciousness" questionnaire, which measures a range of perceptual attributes, including the intensity, vivid-ness, peacefulness, spirituality, and degree of ego dissolution induced by the assigned study intervention.[25] When VR and psilocybin were compared head-to-head, the numerical survey results were nearly superimposable. The Hallucination Machine generated full-fledged STER—that is, a flow state that was selfless, timeless, effortless, and rich. The digital cyberdelic experience was indistinguishable from the pharmacologic psychedelic. Seth proved that his Hallucination Machine was just that—a digital substitute for hallucinogenic mushrooms.

It should come as no surprise that VR is showing promise in exactly the same conditions for which scientists are now testing psychedelics: anxiety, phobias, depression, autism, and PTSD, among other common neuropsychiatric afflictions. In the rest of this chapter, we'll explore how VR is expanding the practice of psychiatry by offering patients a new form of therapy.

Until the late twentieth century, talk therapy was the basis of mental health practice. Pharmaceutical companies then developed effective drug therapies, leading to broad distribution and acceptance of psychoactive medicines like Prozac. When used together, talk therapy and drug therapy can be effective in managing many psychiatric symptoms. But both have their limitations. Talk therapy occurs in the relative comfort and safety of a therapeutic environment, so it's difficult to simulate the real-life circumstances that trigger maladaptive behaviors and thoughts. Patients learn skills in the office, but they still need to practice those skills in the real world. Drug therapy works, too, but the incremental gain is sometimes modest, and side effects are common.

For psychiatrists, VR offers a new digital therapy that does not replace talk or drug therapy, but augments both techniques. In the case of talk therapy, VR allows patients to practice their skills in simulated virtual environments that reflect real-world, stress-inducing scenarios; it offers a safe space to practice and fail without consequences. Lessons learned in the virtual world can transfer to the real world in meaningful and measurable ways. Together with medical and talk therapies, virtual therapy offers a third leg of support. By combining all three types of treatment, psychiatrists have potential to achieve a new level of therapeutic synergy.

I saw this firsthand when I evaluated a patient in the emergency department who got a piece of chicken stuck in his esophagus (expert tip: chew your food carefully). As a gastroenterologist, I'm often called to extricate food that gets lodged in the digestive tract—*somebody's* got to do it. So I went down to the emergency room with my students to meet the patient. We found a young man in great distress. He was beating his chest, sweating profusely, and pacing back and forth like a caged tiger. His behavior seemed out of place for a food impaction, which can certainly be uncomfortable but is not typically a panic-inducing malady once people realize they can breathe and aren't choking. This man could breathe, but something else was the matter.

I asked him to try swallowing some water.

"No way, there's food stuck in my throat. I can't swallow anything."

"I understand, but see if you can swallow just a little bit of water. We're here to help if anything goes wrong."

He gave it a try. Sure enough, the water went down without a problem. There wasn't any chicken stuck in his throat after all. Instead, he was having a full-blown panic attack. The jammed food was not real. Instead, he was experiencing something called globus phenomenon, which is the unsettling, lump-in-the-throat feeling that accompanies extreme anxiety. He was downright panicking. Rather than admit him to the hospital and perform a food disimpaction, I ordered a VR headset to the emergency department. Once it arrived, I dialed up a tranquil beach scene with calming music and asked him to give it a try, which he did.

And then . . . nothing. Absolutely nothing. He sat down and stared straight ahead, completely transfixed, silent, and motionless.

"Feel free to look around. You can explore the scene by moving your head," I said.

Nothing. It was as though he were hypnotized. Two minutes passed without his moving a muscle. It felt like an hour. I started to wonder what was going on inside that headset. Was he asleep? Was he upset? Catatonic? Minutes before he was in the midst of an outright panic attack. There had been a red alert in his brain that something, somewhere, was drastically and existentially wrong. He looked like he was about to die. But now he was calm, still, and quiet.

I decided to remove the headset and reengage. As I lifted the goggles from his face a stream of tears emerged into view. A pool had accumulated under the mask and now, with the dam released, cascaded like a waterfall over his cheeks and mouth.

"Are you okay?"

Silence.

"Everything okay?"

More silence. And then, after a few moments, he awakened from his trance, looked over slowly, and trained his eyes on mine.

"My life is spinning out of control," he said. "My relationships are falling apart. I can't go on like this. I need my life back."

This was as far as I could take him. After all, I'm a gastroenterologist, not a psychiatrist! Within minutes, a VR experience had arrested a full-blown panic attack, prompted a state of tranquility, and generated revelations about his life trajectory. This was not a chicken problem. This was a brain problem—a state of hypervigilance and destructive rumination in need of urgent care. VR cooled his overheated mind by inducing a state of flow. Then, with his mind restored to a calmer state, he was able to self-reflect on what had occurred in a constructive and creative way, yielding new insights that he could not previously access. Rather than admitting him to the hospital, we discharged him from the emergency department in the care of a mental health expert.

Anecdotes can be powerful, but how reproducible is the effect of VR on anxiety? Albert "Skip" Rizzo has been asking this question for most of his academic career. As the director of medical VR at the University of Southern California Institute for Creative Technologies, Rizzo has been a driving force in pioneering VR therapeutics for anxiety. His research is changing lives, one virtual environment at a time.

Classically trained in psychology, Rizzo began his career using traditional talk therapy as the basis of treatment. But over time, he came to realize that talk therapy is limited. "I would sit there for hours talking to patients about their lives, and I knew it helped, but I thought I could do more somehow," he told me. "The problem was that my patients were sitting in an office that bore no resemblance to the places and experiences that caused them distress. An unassuming, bland room is not always conducive to unrooting the causes of mental anguish. I needed to engage my patients in a more compelling and dynamic way. That's when I had my aha moment."

Rizzo's "aha moment" came one day in 1991 when he watched one of his clients playing games on a Nintendo Game Boy. "He wasn't very compliant with my treatment plan," Rizzo said. "But he sure was compliant with that Game Boy. He was utterly transfixed by it! That's when I realized I needed to build some game to help engage my clients in their care. I wasn't yet sure how to do it, but I knew it had to be done."

On that fateful day Rizzo observed pure, unadulterated flow. His client was adrift in the video game environment, where he lost his sense of self, sense of time, and sense of effort. But he knew that first-person shooter games were not designed to treat anxiety. In fact, they might contribute to anxiety in the long run, even if they achieve flow in the short run. Rizzo needed to leverage the entrancing power of games, combine that with the evidence-based principles of talk therapy, and embed the result in a VR headset to bring it all to life.

And that's what he did. Thirty years later, Rizzo has built and tested a range of virtual environments designed to manage anxiety. His most famous program, called *Bravemind*, treats soldiers who are mentally scarred by the calamity of war. By plunging veterans into the thick of battle in a highly realistic virtual environment, Rizzo recreates the visceral, full-body experience of war complete with the bone-rattling vibration of rolling Humvees, the thick scent of burning oil, and the sound of concussive blasts.[26] Through *Bravemind*, Rizzo exposes soldiers to their worst nightmares, but he does it within the controlled safety of VR. His procedure, called VR exposure therapy, gradually inoculates the brain against the triggers of post-traumatic stress disorder. This would normally occur by talking about war, or showing pictures or movies of battle scenes. But

Rizzo found there is no substitute for just *being* in a war. *Bravemind* injects these soldiers right into the front lines, but in a graded, careful manner. When combined with traditional talk therapy and augmented by medical therapy, VR exposure therapy is literally saving lives by rewiring the brain.

Rizzo and his colleagues have published numerous studies using their VR exposure protocols.[27] On average, the treatment works in over two-thirds of patients and the benefits are durable. For example, in one controlled study of VR compared to standard therapy among victims of the World Trade Center attacks—an example applied to a civilian population—a research team led by Barbara Rothbaum and JoAnn Difede worked with Rizzo to show a significant reduction in PTSD symptoms that was maintained six months later.[28] Just like with psychedelics, the benefits persisted well after the treatment period itself, indicating that VR has a sustained impact. In another study, the team found that VR not only lowered psychological symptoms but also reduced physiological measures of startle response and suppressed stress hormones for twelve months after treatment, demonstrating that VR has effects on mind and body.[29] Additional research shows that VR exposure therapy normalizes brain function, which is confirmed on fMRI scans, and that the rewiring persists long after the headsets are removed.[30]

These profound results are now being applied to a range of anxiety disorders and phobias. Studies show that VR exposure therapy can treat arachnophobia, agoraphobia, fear of heights, fear of flying, generalized anxiety disorder, panic disorder, and social anxiety disorder through simulated virtual environments.[31] Although the studies range in size and quality, and despite some variability in results among individual studies, a meta-analysis that combined all the data into one study concluded that VR "is as efficacious as traditional exposure treatment and can be especially useful in the treatment of patients who are resistant to traditional exposure."[32]

Rizzo's research is taking patients beyond the therapist's couch to the site of their original pathology. "We help people to go back to the things that they were traumatized by. We help them to confront those things. To face them. To talk about them. And by this process of doing it repetitively over time, what you see is a gradual decline in the anxiety and the fear response."

Rizzo is showing that VR can profoundly reduce anxiety and change minds for the better, not just by breaking through cycles of unhealthy rumination, but also by carefully reengaging the self-reflective mind to cultivate healthy insights and teach durable skills that help long after the headset is removed.

But beyond calming anticipation anxiety of future events, can VR also manage the self-critical, depressive mind that languishes in the past?

Not long ago, I was asked to evaluate a woman hospitalized with severe depression. Her doctors did not call me to render an opinion about her mood, but rather to sort out why she also had so much abdominal pain. She had experienced recurrent knots in her belly for months, usually in the pit of her stomach just below the breastbone. I looked over her chart and noted the results of several tests. She had already received nearly every lab study, imaging study, and endoscopic study I could think of. The doctors had imaged her body with a CT scan, peered into her stomach with a small camera, and tested for everything from celiac disease to acid reflux. It was all negative.

I decided to offer VR because I sensed her pain might have a mind-body component. My team uses a library with over forty VR experiences, so I asked her what she likes and where she might want to travel. She said she loves the ocean, so we offered her an opportunity to scuba dive with dolphins. She agreed and put on the headset.

At first, she was pleasantly surprised by the realism of the scene. She laughed and smiled. This was a good start. At least she was having fun. But after about five minutes she fell silent. Just total silence, like the panicking man in the emergency room. I've come to learn that silence is okay and not to interrupt. So I stayed with her, for minutes, saying nothing and waiting for a response. She remained still. Her breathing seemed to slow. She was pensive, as if in a hypnotic trance. And then something remarkable happened.

"I figured it out," she said. "I figured out why I have this stomach pain."

"Is that right?"

"Yeah. I figured it out. It's from my brother."

This was unexpected. As far as I knew, she was swimming with dolphins, not relating her abdominal pain to family dynamics. But the virtual environment had caused her to go deep.

"My older brother died of stomach cancer. I think I'm carrying his pain with me."

"But you don't have stomach cancer," I reassured her. "Your tests are negative and the doctors saw nothing in your stomach."

"I know," she replied. "But deep down, I haven't come to terms with his cancer."

She said that she couldn't stop thinking that she, too, had cancer and that the next test would show it. She thought all the previous tests were false negatives, and it was just a matter of time before one came up positive. She said she wasn't yet ready to believe the tests were truly negative.

"But now I know my stomach pain is because of my brother's cancer," she concluded. "I think I'm still mourning his death."

"That's a big breakthrough," I said.

"A year on the couch wouldn't have gotten me here. There's something about these dolphins. They freed me up to think. They helped me figure things out."

Swimming with dolphins was just what she needed to sink into flow, reset her troubled mind, and then arrive at a conceptual breakthrough. With her monkey mind quieted, she was finally able to think deeply and differently. And that benefit—finding headspace to think differently than usual—is a key for managing depression. People need to seek new perspectives outside their own habituated first-person view of the world. That's one reason why talk therapy works, because it allows people to hear objective feedback from a neutral observer and change their perspective for the better.

Chris Brewin, a professor of psychology at the University College London, is taking advantage of VR's view-changing ability to treat depression.

Just like with Mel Slater's research, Brewin uses the principles of embodied cognition to conjure neuro-physical sleight of hand with VR. But instead of simulating an out-of-body experience, he uses VR to embody self-compassion. In a study published by his team in the *British Journal of Psychology*, researchers immersed patients with depression into a virtual body and placed them in a digital living room across from a crying child.[33] They instructed the patients to interact compassionately with the virtual child who was programmed to respond positively to caring gestures. In the next phase of the experiment, the patients were re-embodied within the child and then watched their own recorded compassionate gestures, but this time in reverse from the child's perspective. "By having participants embody an adult and then a child virtual body in succession," lead author Caroline Falconer writes, "our scenario effectively provided a self-to-self situation enabling participants to deliver compassionate sentiments and statements to themselves." The VR program created a radical perspective shift from that of an adult calming a child, to the child being calmed by the adult.

One month after starting the experiment, patients with depression reported a higher sense of self-compassion and a lower degree of self-criticism and depressive symptoms. VR had again quieted the monkey mind. "People with depression with critical internal monologues would not be used to hearing self-directed compassionate statements in their own voice," Brewin writes. "We think that our paradigm furnished individuals with knowledge about the nature and purpose of compassion as well as provided them with a phenomenological experience of giving and receiving it." In other words, Brewin built an empathy machine that boosts positive emotions and combats the self-critical mind by enhancing compassion with self and others.

Back in Professor Slater's lab at the University of Barcelona, I again don a VR headset and enter another of his fantastical worlds. This time I am seated at a table in a modern home with glass walls and spare but well-appointed furnishings. Outside the ceiling-to-floor windows is a sun-dappled lawn bordered by the edge of a forest. It is a peaceful and calm scene. To my left there is a mirror reflecting back my digital avatar.

Prior to entering the virtual environment, Slater had scanned my body to create an exact replica of my face and torso. And sure enough, there I am, freckles and all, looking back in the mirror with a rather serious demeanor.

I am not alone in this room. Sitting across the table is the one and only Daniel Dennett—my undergraduate mentor and renowned philosopher of the mind. I haven't seen him in person for years. He looks considerably older than before, but it's unmistakably Professor Dennett. He is looking back at me, also with a serious demeanor, waiting patiently to engage in dialogue.

This is a jarring experience. Daniel Dennett altered my life in ways he surely never realized. I entered Tufts University in 1990 as a devout theist, and by December of that year was, at best, an agnostic, after trying to square my worldview with his provocative and compelling arguments. In the process of wrestling with his teachings, I learned from Dennett how to think critically using formal logic, how to navigate the intersection between philosophy and science, and how to be a compassionate materialist who views the world with awe through the lens of empiricism. His influence was so great that I formally dedicated one of my medical textbooks to him—a designation he likely doesn't even know about. All of these memories flood back as I sit at this table staring at him in a virtual living room, in a VR headset, in a Barcelona research laboratory, separated in time and space since we last met decades before in his Boston classroom.

It turns out that, unbeknownst to me, Professor Dennett had visited Slater's lab just weeks before my arrival. Slater had scanned his body, too, creating a digital avatar that now sits across from me at the table, ready to talk.

"Go ahead and ask him a question," Slater instructs.

"Okay," I reply. I look Dennett in the eye and pose a question, just like I did thirty years ago in his classroom. "How can I explain consciousness without invoking a God?"

And then . . . I *become* Dennett. I look across the table, and I can see . . . me! We've swapped positions. To my right is a mirror that reflects

Dennett's avatar. I have embodied my own professor. I am now the legend himself. As I stare through Dennett's eyes I see my own freckled face across the table looking back and asking a question.

"How can I explain consciousness without invoking a God?" I hear and see myself ask, but through the ears and eyes of Dennett. Now it's time to respond, but I need to channel the thoughts and voice of Dennett. What would Dennett say? I think about it for a second and then reply:

"Why do you need to invoke a God? I don't understand why that even matters," I say through the personage of Dennett.

And now I am back in my own body, listening to Dennett say what I just said, yet in his own voice, not in mine. The software has permuted my voice to sound like his voice—the same voice you'll hear in his TED talks, but with my words coming out of his mouth. I listen in my restored first-person perspective as Dennett repeats my response.

And back and forth we go. For several minutes we spar about the nature of consciousness, dualism, materialism, and other Philosophy 101 topics we debated decades before. Once again, Dennett has won the debate, although I beat myself through his avatar in a twisted, ego-dissolving virtual exchange. I say ego-dissolving not only because I lose the philosophical argument (ego bruised again by Dennett), but also because I once again feel my selfhood distributed beyond my corporeal boundaries. My consciousness is allocated between two bodies, just as it had been in the earlier out-of-body experience. I remove the VR headset and return to the real world, convinced that I still cannot dismiss Dennett's worldview. Using Dennett as my alter ego, Slater had engaged me in self-dialogue with my influential mentor, enabling a sort of self-counseling session.*

My encounter with Dennett suggests that VR could offer self-counseling for other topics beyond the academic concerns of a former philosophy major. Could this technique also expand the client-therapist relationship for talk therapy? Traditionally, therapists and clients sit face-to-face. With VR, clients could meet their therapist from anywhere in

---

* You can watch the entire six-minute exchange between me and myself (as Dennett) at this website: www.virtualmedicine.health/dennett.

the world through virtual telecounseling. They might view each other's avatar in tailored therapeutic environments. Someone with alcohol use disorder might hold a session in a bar, triggering brainstem cravings not otherwise possible during typical therapy. A client suffering from depression might sit on a beach in Big Sur, transfixed by gorgeous scenery while learning the techniques of mindful meditation. And people might not only meet with their real therapists but also select any virtual therapist they could imagine like, say, Sigmund Freud.

Leave it to Mel Slater to have already covered that ground. In another pioneering study by his team, titled "Conversations Between Self and Self as Sigmund Freud—A Virtual Body Ownership Paradigm for Self Counselling," Slater invited people to discuss their mental health issues directly with Freud.[34] In the experiment, participants entered a virtual environment similar to what I experienced with Dennett, but rather than encountering a former professor, there was Freud himself, ready to assist. The research subjects described a personal problem to Freud, switched roles, and then offered counseling back to themselves through Freud's persona. These conversations were often extensive, as people worked through their issues with the assistance of Freud's virtual presence. For example, one participant explained to his Freud counselor that he deeply missed a girl he had been close with but who had moved away to study elsewhere. Embodied as Freud, he replied:

> Well, I recommend you move on because it doesn't really solve anything. It's not a huge problem, but it doesn't help to live in the past. I think you should keep it as a good experience and memory, but not something that keeps you from going on.

The participant again switched back into his own persona and reflected on Freud's advice:

> It's true, it's very true I shouldn't be living in the past. You can miss someone a lot, but it doesn't have to be something that keeps you from going on, from living your life and living the moment, you know,

everyone follows his own path and you have to meet new people that gives you something else. You have to live every day at the maximum, enjoying life.[35]

Slater found that people reported significant improvements in their mood and happiness when they underwent self-counseling with Freud. In contrast, a control group who spoke to avatars of themselves did not feel better; only talking with Freud did the trick of breaking out of the cognitive rut. "This suggests that embodied perspective taking can lead to sufficient detachment from habitual ways of thinking about personal problems," Slater concluded.[36]

Virtual self-counseling holds promise for healing by leveraging our natural inclination for inner dialogue, but in a constructive and supportive way. In contrast to the unhealthy ruminating mind, where people become too invested in their first-person narratives about the world, Slater's technique offers mental space for alternative interpretations. The key is to break the cycle of self-talk by introducing an intermediary, even if that intermediary is the self, virtually embodied in the shell of another.

Whether it's lying on a beach in the emergency department to arrest a panic attack, swimming with dolphins in the hospital to treat depression, revisiting the atrocities of war to combat PTSD, or communing with Sigmund Freud to manage relationships, these stories teach us how to go beyond the therapist's couch and into therapeutic worlds previously inaccessible, if not unimaginable.

CHAPTER THREE

Creating a Distraction

E RIN MARTUCCI HAS JUST BEEN HANDED A VR HEADSET. A FORTY-year-old mother of a young child, Erin is now in the midst of delivering her second baby at Orange Regional Medical Center in New Jersey, and the contractions are starting to get intense.

"Give this a try," says her obstetrician, Ralph Anderson, who notices that Erin is beginning to struggle. Dr. Anderson knows that Erin wants to avoid a spinal injection to dull the pain. She previously used an epidural during the birth of her first child but regretted how long it took for her infant to bond and breastfeed after the delivery because of side effects from the pain medicine. In her pre-labor planning this time around, Erin explained that she wanted a natural birth.

Still, virtual reality may not have been what Erin had in mind. She regards the headset quizzically. "I feel terrible saying this, Dr. Anderson, but I don't think this is gonna help. I'm teetering on the edge."

"Why not give it a shot?" asks her husband. "If you don't like it, then you can always take it off."

"Okay, I've got nothing to lose," she says. Erin rides out a contraction, catches her breath, and slides on the headset.

She is now seated by a campfire in the middle of a pastel-hued, sparkling forest. Erin is immersed in ethereal, rhythmic music that aligns with her breathing, as if she is conducting a techno-symphony with her own diaphragm. As Erin breathes in, and out, in, and out, concentric circles expand and contract around the campfire in synchrony. When she exhales, a stream of effervescent sparks flow out of her mouth and into the campfire. Fireflies flit about the scene. Clouds of lavender and blue vapor seep out from behind nearby stones, lending an otherworldly, almost psychedelic quality to the pulsating landscape.

She is completely immersed in the scene. The birthing room has been replaced by a wondrous and colorful world; her mind is fully occupied. Erin's sense of self, which moments before was girding against waves of pain, is now spread about the digital equivalent of a Monet watercolor. A woman with a British accent begins to speak. With a calm and steady demeanor, the voice coaches Erin through Lamaze breathing.

Two hours have passed when Dr. Anderson interrupts: "Okay, Erin, you're ready to push."

"What?"

"It's time to have your baby. Her head is coming out."

Erin has lost her sense of time; she is stunned by the stark interruption. Dr. Anderson removes the headset, reintroducing her to the sights and sounds of childbirth. Her baby girl is crowning. Erin delivers within less than a minute.

Her newborn daughter, Elizabeth, awakens to her own abrupt shift in reality. She locks eyes with her mom and then begins to breastfeed. And with that, Elizabeth becomes the first baby documented to enter real reality with the help of virtual reality.[1]

In this chapter, we discover why Erin was able to deliver her baby without an epidural, and more generally, how immersive therapeutics manage physical pain. This includes not just childbirth, but conditions ranging from burn injuries to fibromyalgia to irritable bowel syndrome.

Immersion alleviates these conditions through its second therapeutic mechanism: dampening inner pain signals.

VR lowers the perception of pain in at least three different ways. First, it distracts the brain from noxious signals rising up from the body. Second, it creates an illusion of time acceleration, effectively shortening the length of pain episodes. And third, it nips signals in the bud at their origin, blocking pain from reaching the brain. The combination of these effects supports the ability of immersion to fight pain.

Let's begin with the first effect of distracting the brain from pain. An exercise will help. How many times have you blinked in the last minute? How many breaths have you taken? How many times has your heart beat since you started this chapter? If you are sitting on a chair or lying on a bed or couch, have you noticed the pressure of that surface pressing back against your body, keeping you from falling to the ground? What does your scalp feel like right now? Can you sense your clothes rubbing against your body, or feel the paper or e-reader in your hands?

Maybe you can now. But I'm guessing if so, it's only because I posed the questions. Sorry about that. Keeping track of eye blinks, buttocks pressure, or breaths can be a bit maddening.

Our brains are not designed to pay attention to peripheral phenomena while attending to other, more engaging tasks. As a result, we become blind to phenomena outside our spotlight of attention. This is called inattentional blindness. Perhaps the most famous example of inattentional blindness is the "invisible gorilla" effect, based on an ingenious experiment developed by Christopher Chabris and Daniel Simons. In the experiment, you watch a video of six people passing a basketball back and forth.[2] (See the Notes and References section for a link to the video.) Three of the players are wearing white shirts and three are wearing black shirts. The task is simple: count how many times the white-shirted players pass the ball. The answer is fifteen times. Most people get that right. But about half the viewers completely miss the tall figure in a gorilla suit who traipses into the middle of the scene, vigorously beats its chest, and nonchalantly walks off. This is an astounding demonstration of our tendency to miss obvious phenomena, especially when we're engaged in complex tasks. Our conscious self becomes easily distracted and misses things—even big, hairy, chest-beating gorillas. Now that you know the trick, it will be hard for you to miss the gorilla when you watch the video. The research team prepared a second video for people who have already watched the first video. (You'll find a link to that video in the Notes and References section of this book. See if you can detect the obvious changes in their second video.)[3]

The invisible gorilla experiment isn't really fair. After all, we are not prepared to see a gorilla, we weren't asked to see a gorilla, and we would never *expect* to see a gorilla. So why should someone watching the video expect a gorilla to casually walk through the scene? It's not at all equivalent to Erin Martucci's delivery; we would fully expect Erin to focus intensely on her labor pain because it's too prominent to ignore.

Another team at Harvard modified the gorilla experiment to make it a little more fair to the research subjects. They decided to study a group of radiologists because these doctors are trained to inspect images carefully, find intricate patterns in radiographs, and make life-or-death decisions on the basis of their review.[4] Would radiologists miss the gorilla?

The researchers took a photo of a man in a gorilla suit, shrunk it down to the size of a matchbook, and then spliced the mini ape into real images being reviewed by radiologists. Moreover, the researchers instructed the man in the gorilla suit to "shake his hand angrily" for the photo. This was not just a mini gorilla—it was an *angry* mini gorilla. The doctors were not informed about the experiment and went about their business reading the scan as they normally would. Surely, trained radiologists—*professional lookers*—wouldn't miss a fierce hairy creature sitting in the middle of a CT scan image.

Eighty-three percent of the radiologists completely missed the gorilla hiding in plain sight. Surely the radiologists *saw* the gorillas. Their eyes met the photons emanating from the angry gorilla man—but their brains did not register the information reaching their eyes. There was an utter disconnect. The radiologists' brains were prepared to see what they were prepared to see, and not much else. They were focused on looking for other things, like tumors, infections, or abnormal patterns in the lungs, heart, and blood vessels. There was too much else to investigate. The attention circuits in the brain were preoccupied by scanning for pixelated patterns of disease but were not prepared, or even able, to find the gorilla. It's not that the radiologists were failing to pay attention. It's that they were *paying very close attention*—laser focused attention, even—on the stuff that mattered most.

When neuroscientists and psychologists refer to inattentional blindness, they don't just mean blindness to visual objects before our eyes but also to the "blindness" of our other senses (smells, sounds, tastes, and others), and even our "blindness" to more complex phenomena such as behaviors and emotions, both in ourselves and in others. Understanding the neuropsychology of this human shortcoming helps us understand how VR distracts the brain from pain. It all works according to the same basic logic of how and why our brains choose what to pay attention to.

Start by focusing your mind on something mundane. Stop reading for a second and listen. *Really listen.* What ambient noise do you hear right now? Are there people talking around you? Cars outside a window? An air vent blowing? Music? Whatever you hear, just focus all your attention on it. If you hear nothing, then regard the sound of silence. Even then you should hear your heart beating or your breathing. Try to put down this book and listen for as long as you can. Try to sense as much nuance and detail as you're able.

How did you do? How long were you able to sustain your attention? Some of you made a conscious decision not to even try, instead opting to read on and just get to the point of this exercise. Some of you gave it a try, perhaps for ten seconds, perhaps for longer, and maybe you took notice of some sounds and regarded them briefly. Others may have stayed with it for longer still, perhaps noticing the unexpected rhythms of your acoustic environment, maybe even wondering how you failed to register all that sound before tuning in. But no matter how you conducted this exercise, all of you eventually came back to reading this book. At some point, your brain made an executive decision: time to stop listening and start reading again.

This exercise demonstrates a fundamental ability we often take for granted: the ability to manipulate our attention. Under normal circumstances, it is not difficult for us to shift our attention from one object to another. In fact, it is surprisingly easy to flip our attention at will; perhaps it's *too* easy, as most of us know from surfing the internet or incessantly checking social media. Stimuli constantly compete for our attention. When your attention is temporarily drawn away from its target, we call it a distraction. If the distraction causes you to switch to a new task altogether, then we call it a more sustained interruption.[5]

Right now these words have your attention. You are reading them and regarding them. The ambient noise has shifted to the background for the moment. You have made a conscious choice to continue reading rather than actively listening. Your eardrums are still vibrating from pressure waves, and your eighth cranial nerve—the nerve that transmits sounds to your brain—is still firing away, dutifully sending its signals to a cerebral waystation for processing. But your brain is too busy reading to register and interpret the arrival of those signals. The spotlight of your attention is focused on reading.

This would imply that multitasking as we understand it is a myth. We cannot effectively attend to multiple tasks at once, even if we think we can. Instead, we engage in task shifting, meaning we select one task over another, and then switch back and forth to work on multiple tasks serially, but not at the exact same time.[6] Although we might perceive this frenetic shifting as multitasking and convince ourselves that we can parallel process, it is more accurate to call this continuous partial attention, a term coined by former Microsoft executive Linda Stone, who observed that our perception of continuous multitasking is really a consequence of doing multiple things poorly by switching back and forth without sustained attention.[7]

But we *can* sustain our attention on one task at a time. Consider what happened when I asked you to focus on the noises around you. In that moment, you placed more emphasis on the ambient sounds, causing it to swing your attention toward listening. At the same time, you placed less emphasis on reading. It's not just that you focused more on sound, *it's also that you focused less on reading,* so as to make doubly sure you would attend to listening. This distinction is important, because it reflects two processes that occur in tandem. The heavier emphasis on listening resulted from an effect called selective attention, and the lighter emphasis on reading resulted from selective ignoring. Understanding the difference is crucial to understand how VR combats pain.

The dual processes of attending and ignoring carve the lens that focuses our attention spotlight. Whereas selective attention directs our spotlight toward the task at hand, selective ignoring prevents us from looking away by keeping irrelevant stimuli in the dark. The net effect is enhanced perceptual contrast—that is, a sharp spotlight. This is the essence of what's known as the spotlight theory of attention.

Adam Gazzaley's lab at the University of California, San Francisco, has for years been studying the cognitive yin and yang of attending and ignoring. In one experiment, his team exposed research subjects to a series of pictures, some of people's faces and others of nature scenes.[8] First, they asked the participants to passively take in the images without any instructions. Then they instructed participants to actively remember some, but not all, of the images. Sometimes they told the research subjects to remember the faces and to ignore the nature scenes. Other times, they said to remember only the nature scenes and to ignore the faces. Then, after a brief delay, the participants had to recall the memorized images. All the while, the research subjects were lying in an fMRI scanner that took pictures of their brain activity.

Gazzaley found that when subjects passively viewed the images without instruction, the vision circuits in their brain perked up a little bit on the fMRI, but not a lot. That wasn't too surprising. Next, he observed that when subjects memorized images, their brain circuits lighted up even more than at baseline. He called this neural enhancement. But perhaps most surprising, Gazzaley revealed that when subjects viewed the irrelevant images, their brain circuits dimmed down below baseline levels, denoting an active process of forgetting. He called this neural suppression. Gazzaley writes that "what we learned from this experiment was that the act of ignoring is not a passive process; rather, the goal to ignore something is an active one." Neural suppression, he explains, decreases the noise and lets the signal shine. "Although it may seem counterintuitive, we now appreciate that focusing and ignoring are *not* two sides of the same coin . . . they are two separate coins."[9]

Gazzaley's work explains why radiologists miss the gorilla in the CT scan. Inattentional blindness is the result of neural suppression—it is an active, resource-consuming process that augments our ability to focus attention selectively. The radiologists miss the gorilla precisely because they are focusing so hard on everything else that matters while suppressing the irrelevant gorilla pixels.

When Erin was in labor, she was focused on the task of delivering her daughter. She experienced powerful contractions and expressed concern that she might require an epidural to manage the pain. If Dr. Anderson had instructed Erin simply to focus on the ambient noise of the delivery room as a countermeasure to her worsening labor pain, it probably wouldn't have worked. Listening to ambient noise is not a compelling, vivid, or arresting experience on par with childbirth. Swinging the attention spotlight away from an intense experience like labor requires a counter-distraction of even greater sensory magnitude than the labor itself. That's a tall order.

The human brain does a lot of things, but it is especially well engineered to create the sense of vision. Nearly one-third of the brain's cortex—the outer shell devoted to thinking, moving, and sensing—is composed of hundreds of millions of neurons that support vision. In contrast, only 8 percent of the cortex is devoted to touch, and even less—a measly 3 percent—is dedicated to hearing.[10] When we are awake and our eyes are open, about two-thirds of the electrical activity in our brain is related to visual processing, yielding an astounding three billion neuronal firings *per second*. There are more neurons dedicated to vision than to the four other basic senses combined (touch, taste, smell, and hearing). This emphasis on sight makes evolutionary sense, because long before our ancestors were reading and writing, they were watching prey across vast plains, or peering carefully through dense forests for subtle signs of trouble. Of course, they also used touch, smell, taste, and hearing to make sense of the world. But there's nothing like *seeing* a tiger coming at you to prepare a defense—the speed of light is much faster than the speed of sound, and by the time you can smell or feel a tiger, well, it's probably too late.

The sheer amount of brain power dedicated to vision means that if you want to distract someone, there's no better way to do it than by manipulating what they see. Bombard the eyes with spectacular and dynamic visions, and next thing you know, those three billion neuronal firings per second will ricochet through half the brain to process the overwhelming load of visual data.

This is why virtual reality is so good at managing pain. What better way to deliver a nearly inconceivable amount of data points, in so little time, than to immerse the brain in a three-dimensional world of brilliant, glimmering images. By introducing an immersive, vivid, unexpected, 360-degree visualization, Dr. Anderson directed Erin's prefrontal cortex to take notice, draw down neural bandwidth from other sensory networks, and shift its attention from labor pain to a new virtual world.

There was a gorilla right in Erin's view, but she couldn't see it.

So far, we have discussed the first of three effects that allow VR to dampen inner pain signals: distracting the brain through inattentional blindness. Depending on the strength and frequency of the pain signals, VR may have an easier or harder time running interference. When pain is severe, chances are that distraction alone won't be enough. This brings us to the second beneficial effect of VR on pain: time acceleration.

Recall that Erin was shocked to learn that two hours had passed when Dr. Anderson tapped on her shoulder and told her to push. When I spoke to Erin afterward, she said the two hours "flew by," as if time itself had accelerated. She said the two hours felt, at most, like only thirty minutes. Why is that?

The answer has something to do with working memory, which refers to the part of short-term memory that temporarily stores information in our mind's eye after its source has disappeared from view.[11] For example, if you close your eyes, can you still picture the environment around you? Can you imagine the details of what is behind you, or above you, without taking a peek? Your brain is constantly tracking the sights, smells, sounds, and feelings of your environment. This ability is critical for engaging in everyday life, because without working memory, you would lose track of conversations, forget where you are, and become disassociated from your physical environment. Research also shows that working memory is important for keeping track of time.[12]

It turns out that working memory is, once again, controlled by the prefrontal cortex. Maintaining information in short-term memory is an active process that requires the prefrontal cortex to expend neural energy. Working memory engages the same selective attention networks that activate when the object in memory is present in reality. Normally, we have enough bandwidth to support the prefrontal cortex in recording short-term events. But when the brain is occupied, its working memory is impeded and funny stuff can happen. You can lose track of time, or you can become disassociated from your surroundings (like the "highway hypnosis" we discussed in Chapter 2). Disassociated living is not adaptive under normal circumstances, but it can be highly adaptive when you are attempting to escape a painful reality.

Gazzaley's team investigated what happens to working memory under experimental conditions. In a series of carefully controlled studies, his team found that working memory is undermined when the brain confronts visual stimulation.[13] The more complex the visualization, the harder it becomes to bolster short-term memory. This is not just a matter of keeping your eyes open or closed; it is a function of the image itself. For example, staring into a gray screen does not impact your working memory, but staring at a nature scene does. The busier the scene, the harder it is to maintain working memory. When Gazzaley studied the brain directly using fMRI scans, he found that visual distraction undermined the prefrontal cortex and affected the brain structures devoted to memory storage. Moreover, when his team disrupted the prefrontal cortex using a special magnet placed over the forehead, they discovered that short-term memory was dramatically impacted. The prefrontal cortex could no longer filter out distractions, leaving the brain bewildered because it was without the stabilizing ballast of working memory.

In this way, VR occupied Erin's prefrontal cortex. Unable to keep track of moment-to-moment events in real reality, she lost track of the birthing process, and instead entrained her mind on the virtual scene. Time contracted. Erin became disassociated from reality in a dreamlike, time warping, virtual world that not only tipped her attention away from labor pains but also convinced her mind that the experience was happening faster than its actual duration.

Imagine if we had a fast-forward button for the painful moments in our lives. For Erin, VR was that button. But how well does VR work for other people? How reproducible is this effect?

The illusion of VR time acceleration has also been demonstrated in clinical research. In a 2012 study from Mashhad University of Medical Sciences in Iran, a research team assessed the effect of VR during episiotomy repair after labor and delivery.[14] Some challenging deliveries require a surgical incision to aid passage of the baby's head. This procedure is called an episiotomy. The incision is repaired with sutures shortly after childbirth. Although obstetricians inject anesthetics into the area prior to closing the surgical cut, the procedure can still be painful. The researchers wanted to see if VR could help with pain management. They randomly separated a group of thirty women requiring episiotomy into two equal groups: one received VR during the surgical closure, the other did not. Both groups received standard local anesthesia with lidocaine, a numbing medicine that helps lower pain in the immediate area but does not enter the bloodstream or reach the brain. The VR intervention was an underwater scene of dolphins and whales using a 3-D video produced by IMAX.

The researchers measured pain during the episiotomy to see if there were any differences between groups. During the procedure, severe pain was reported in 60 percent of women in the control group despite receiving the local anesthesia, whereas only 20 percent of the VR group experienced severe pain. That's a difference of 40 percent, which in medical studies is a very large clinical effect size. Also, patients in the VR group perceived that the repair took *46 percent less time* than the actual duration of the procedure. Similar to Erin's experience of time acceleration during her labor, patients in this study sensed a similar VR-induced time warp.

Investigators in the United States have documented similar benefits in obstetrics. In a 2018 study conducted at the University of Michigan and supported by the National Institutes of Health, a team of obstetricians and anesthesiologists led by David Frey investigated the use of VR in a group of laboring women.[15] The study was limited to patients giving birth for the first time who were early in labor but who had not yet requested an epidural injection. Dr. Frey randomized the women into two groups: one group started with VR for a period of time, but then stopped using VR and continued laboring without the headset. The second group reversed the order by starting without VR for a while, and then donned the headset. After each interval, the patients completed questionnaires to measure pain, anxiety, nausea, and perception of the VR experience. Rather than sitting in a psychedelic dream forest, the women in this study all watched "curious manatees" in a scuba diving simulation while listening to "nighttime sleep music" that overlaid the sounds of manatee calls and breathing underwater. As an aside, our team also uses underwater VR scenes on occasion. We've found that some patients love it, but some don't. For some people, being underwater feels more oppressive and threatening than whatever they were experiencing before entering VR. It is important to ask patients about aquaphobia before dunking them underwater!

What did the researchers find? Not only were pain scores lower during the VR treatment periods, but VR also caused patients to spend less time ruminating about their pain and to experience less anxiety, compared to periods without VR. Eighty-two percent reported that they either "very much" or "completely" enjoyed using VR during labor. Importantly, the investigators observed no adverse events from the VR, and there was no worsening of nausea while bobbing underwater with the manatees.

These clinical trials indicate that Erin's story is not unique. In an even larger VR childbirth study led by Drs. Melissa Wong and Kim

Gregory, our research team at Cedars-Sinai found similar results as the University of Michigan study.[16] There is now sufficient data to say that VR is a viable and safe option for pain management during labor and delivery. Given the favorable risk-benefit ratio of VR, it seems reasonable for obstetric wards to offer headsets early and often as a drug-free alternative—or at least as a therapeutic adjunct—to standard anesthesia.

Dr. Anderson and Erin Martucci were clearly onto something. Decades before them, a duo of pioneering psychologists at the University of Washington named Hunter Hoffman and David Patterson had an early hunch that VR could treat severe pain, not just from normal physiologic events like childbirth but also for painful diseases. They had studied the evidence that drug-free distractions such as meditation, music therapy, humor therapy, and watching movies could all modify pain perception, and they wondered if VR could do the same. Hoffman and Patterson were heavily influenced by the theoretical underpinnings of another pair of scientists, Ronald Melzack and Patrick Wall, who in 1965 proposed the revolutionary gate control theory of pain.[17] It's worth spending a few moments to review this groundbreaking theory because it expands our understanding of how VR operates on the nervous system, and it introduces the third method by which VR dampens pain: blocking signals from reaching the brain.

Prior to 1965, when Melzack and Wall described their gate control theory in the journal *Science*, pain was considered to be a simple bell-ringing alarm system that warned the body of injury. This concept, originally described by Descartes in 1644, asserted that pain was transmitted along a one-way street from its source to the brain.[18] It turned out this was yet another thing Descartes got wrong. But for over three hundred years, the Cartesian notion of pain as a one-way street was propagated as gospel, until Melzack and Wall proposed a more nuanced, interesting, and evidence-based model.

They argued that pain signals travel through a transmission station in the spinal cord that determines whether and how fast the signals rise up into the brain. They explained that before pain signals can shoot up the spinal cord, they first have to pass through a "gate" that is either opened or closed. If the gate is closed, then the pain gets held up and may never make it up to the brain. If the gate is open, then the pain signals pass through the checkpoint and are free to ascend the spinal cord to the brain. Everything we discussed before about the prefrontal cortex, attention spotlight, VR time acceleration, and so forth, assumes that pain signals enter the brain in the first place. But if the signals never arrive in the brain, then none of that matters; the brain has nothing to process if the signals are jammed up along the interoceptive highway.

The gate control theory went a step further. Melzack and Wall showed that pain gates can be opened or closed by the brain itself. They revealed that pain is not solely transmitted along an ascending pathway from the site of injury to the brain, but that pain is also affected by a descending pathway originating in the brain that can open or close the gates in the spinal cord. *This was a massive breakthrough, because it meant that what happens in our mind can govern how pain is transmitted from the far reaches of our body.*

The gate control theory proposed that physical, emotional, and social factors govern whether the pain gates are open or closed. For example, feeling relaxed or upbeat, or just being distracted, can send signals from the brain down the spinal cord to close the pain gates. It's as if the brain is saying to the body, "I'm doing well right now, thank you, so no need to bother me with any pain. Keep it to yourself!" In contrast, feeling upset, fearful, or anxious can send signals downstream to *open* the gates, triggering a vicious cycle of accelerated pain perception. It's as if the hypervigilant brain is saying, "I'm really on edge, so I need to know if anything bad is going on down there." In short, the gate control theory proposed that the brain is not just a hapless recipient of pain signals, but that it actively controls which signals it receives in the first place.

This brings us back to Hoffman and Patterson, who were in graduate school obtaining their respective PhDs in psychology in an era when gate control theory was finally becoming accepted as scientific dogma (it took over a decade after the *Science* article before Descartes's hold on the field was finally shaken). Hoffman had expertise in a wide range of areas that included memory, the phenomenon of magical thinking, and even bioelectromagnetics. Patterson was a clinical psychologist with expertise in hypnosis, rehabilitation medicine, and pain. Inspired by the work of Melzack and Wall, they combined their diverse interests to co-originate what is now called VR analgesia, the technical term for VR pain treatment. Their foundational research set the stage for Erin Martucci and thousands of other patients who use VR for pain today.

Hoffman and Patterson tested the pain-fighting benefits of VR through a series of rigorous experiments over decades of careful analysis. Although they did not study the use of VR during childbirth, they evaluated the impact of VR on patients with another type of intense pain: severe burn injuries. There are few sensory experiences more excruciating than an extensive burn. Worse still, when patients are managed in specialized burn units, they are subjected to agonizing bandage changes to help promote healing. In a paradoxical way, peeling away damaged skin allows it to heal. Yet at the same time, the skin stiffens and scars, so patients need to stretch back the skin through a physical therapy process that causes searing pain. It's hard to imagine anything more intense.

The pain of burn injuries is typically managed with a cocktail of strong opioid medications. Pills such as hydrocodone (Vicodin) and oxycodone (Percocet) are often used to manage background pain, and then intravenous or injectable opioids such as morphine and hydromorphone (Dilaudid) are administered during acutely painful episodes like bandage changes and wound cleaning. These medicines can be powerful analgesics, but they have serious side effects (more on that in Chapter 7) and, over time, lead to tolerance after repeated uses. Opioids eventually lose their effect, leaving patients desperate for another remedy to soothe their pain, while, at the same time, making them physically and emotionally dependent on their failing medical regimen.

Hoffman and Patterson thought there had to be a better way. Combining the spotlight theory of attention with gate control theory, they devised a specialized VR treatment for burn injuries called *SnowWorld*.[19] Their brilliant idea was to counterbalance the searing pain of a burn with the cool, soothing sensation of being in a wintry scene. They hypothe-sized that VR could both distract the brain from arriving pain signals (the spotlight theory) *and* nip signals in the bud before they even arrived in the brain (the gate control theory). In *SnowWorld*, patients score points by tossing virtual snowballs at penguins, snowmen, and igloos perched along snow-covered cliffs and canyons while listening to, of all things, "You Can Call Me Al" by Paul Simon (from the album *Graceland*, one of my favorites). Developed in the year 2000, *SnowWorld* was way ahead of its time in terms of graphics, user immersion, and sense of presence.

A series of uncontrolled studies revealed profound pain-reduction benefits from *SnowWorld*. Hoffman and Patterson then subjected their game to a formal randomized controlled trial.[20] In their 2011 study con-ducted at the University of Washington Regional Burn Center at the Harborview Medical Center in Seattle, the research team recruited chil-dren and young adults who required physical therapy to treat severe burn injuries. They randomized patients into VR and non-VR usage periods and compared pain reports between conditions.

The results were again dramatic. *SnowWorld* reduced cognitive pain by 44 percent, emotional pain by 32 percent, and sensory pain by 27 per-cent. They also asked patients how much "fun" they had during physical therapy for their burns, which is a curious question for such a punishing experience. Patients reported a threefold increase in "fun" while in VR. It is telling that patients would have any fun at all while having their burns stretched and manipulated, much less three times as much enjoy-ment while in VR. This highlights the level of immersion achieved in *SnowWorld* and its powerful ability to control attention by running neural interference. Notably, the benefits of VR did not wane over repeated use, indicating persistent benefits beyond the first treatment period. The au-thors also reported that the effect was more pronounced in patients who felt most immersed in the experience, revealing a dose-response relation-ship between the degree of presence and the amount of pain reduction.

The University of Washington team conducted another key experi-ment to evaluate brain activity in patients using VR.[21] They created a cus-tom "magnet-friendly" headset that could be safely used within an fMRI machine (the fMRI uses a big magnet that can damage some equipment). Then they asked normal control subjects to wear the VR goggles, enter the machine, and sustain thirty seconds of a hot probe applied to their feet, followed by another thirty seconds of a lukewarm temperature as a non-pain control. The hot probe was pretty hot—not bad enough to cause damage, but no fun, either. Finally, the scientists watched brain activity on the fMRI scan to see if anything changed while the subjects experienced pain in VR as compared to not being in VR.

They found that pain was again mitigated by VR. That part was not surprising. But this time around, they confirmed that VR has direct effects on the brain. When Hoffman and Patterson compared brain scans with VR versus without VR, they discovered a 50 percent reduction in activity across multiple brain regions associated with pain. Not only was activity lower in the brain's cortex, where pain signals coming up from the spinal cord are received and processed, but activity was also lower in the insula, which is part of the limbic system that handles the emotional aspects of pain. In other words, this critical study demonstrated that VR not only tamps down the sensation of pain, but it also curtails the negative emotions and cognitions associated with the pain. This was a fundamental breakthrough.

Inspired by the work of Hoffman and Patterson, researchers around the world have now studied VR analgesia for a wide range of acute pain conditions. Some studies use VR to test the reduction of pain for dental procedures, spinal taps, urological procedures, colonoscopies, chemotherapy infusions, and intravenous needle sticks.[22] There is even evidence that VR helps reduce chronic itchiness from atopic dermatitis and psoriasis.[23]

In 2018, a research team from Monash Medical Centre in Australia published a meta-analysis—a study of studies—of randomized VR pain trials.[24] After crunching the numbers across studies from around the world, they concluded that VR is indeed better than control conditions for managing acute pain, although they observed that the quality of many VR trials is lacking and emphasized that more rigorous studies are needed to advance the field. I will return to this issue in Chapter 9 where we discuss how to standardize high-quality VR treatment trials.

Overall, the weight of the evidence shows that VR provides meaningful benefits for acute pain, whether it be for labor pain, burn pain, dental pain, procedural pain, or postsurgical pain. Hoffman and Patterson have shown that VR directly affects the brain and combats pain at the extremes of human tolerance.

Up to this point we've focused on how VR improves somatic pain, which is the type of pain that comes from muscles, bones, tendons, skin, and soft tissues in the body. But there is another type of pain we haven't yet discussed: visceral pain. This is the type of pain that arises from the inner organs, including the lungs, heart, urinary system, and digestive system. Whereas somatic pain can be pinpointed to a specific area of the body, visceral pain often feels diffuse and can even radiate to far reaches of the body that are well beyond the site of disease. The pain is experienced differently because somatic and visceral pain travel to the brain along different pathways, with visceral pain taking a more circuitous and tangled route than somatic pain. Nonetheless, both somatic and visceral pain are experienced in the brain, meaning it is possible that VR's effects on the brain could treat both types of pain.

As a gastroenterologist, I have a special interest in visceral pain from the abdominal organs. The gastrointestinal system is constantly churning, grinding, and secreting substances. These are normally unconscious events, but when things go wrong in the digestive tract it can lead to bothersome symptoms. Irritable bowel syndrome (IBS), inflammatory bowel disease, acid reflux disease, and celiac disease are examples of common visceral pain conditions. People with these diseases may experience stomach pain, cramping, bloating, and other uncomfortable sensations in the belly. Can immersive therapeutics help these types of visceral pain? I thought it was worth a try.

The first time I tested VR for visceral pain was with an IBS patient who had severe abdominal pain that required hospitalization and intravenous morphine. She had received many previous therapies, from antibiotics to strong medicines that alter gut contractions, but nothing seemed to work. The morphine wasn't working either, so her doctors escalated therapy and added a drug called ketamine, a powerful medicine that lulls patients into a trance-like psychedelic state. That also didn't work. The doctors called my team to see if we could offer any other treatments. They were surprised when we suggested VR. We placed her in a relaxing virtual environment with waterfalls and meadows, and then we waited to see what would happen next. Within ten minutes of using VR she reported "zero pain." She literally said, "I'm ready to go home, as long as I can bring this thing with me." She was discharged the next day after nearly a week in the hospital. I checked on her a couple days later and she said the pain was still diminished and she wasn't using any meds. This was a dramatic response. VR is by no means a miracle cure (more on this in Part II), but her experience revealed to me that VR can help with visceral pain and may continue to work even after the headset is removed.

Just how does VR help with visceral pain conditions like IBS? And is the effect reproducible with other patients? To answer these questions, we need to discuss how the brain and gut communicate.

You already know the brain and the gut must be connected. If you've ever felt "nervous" in the belly, say, before giving a big speech or launching into a business pitch, then you know the bowels keep close tabs on the brain. If you've ever taken a final exam, maybe you felt some anxiety just before the test . . . maybe you even raced to the bathroom with diarrhea. Or if you've ever had bacterial food poisoning, then you know your belly is alerted to the intruder before your conscious brain has any clue (and your brain has probably never forgotten the visceral anguish wrought by the gut).

But even more than that, the brain and gut are physically and chemically inseparable. We call this the brain-gut axis. If you were exploring a jungle ten thousand years ago and heard a tiger roar, you'd probably have felt a sharp pang in your abdomen. You might have felt "butterflies," queasiness, or outright nausea. Your gut would have informed you, quite literally, that a threat was lurking nearby. You'd have either fought the tiger or run away in panic: the classic fight or flight response. And here you are now, reading this book, because tigers did not eat your ancestors. At least, they didn't eat them as quickly as they ate other people's ancestors. And I am here now, typing these words, because my ancestors also had gut feelings that kept them a step ahead of predators, human or otherwise. We are all here because our predecessors had fantastic visceral sensors.

The bowels usually tell the brain what to do—not the other way around. The main interoceptive link between the brain and the gut, called the vagus nerve, has ten times more fibers running from the gut to the brain than vice versa.[25] Scientists refer to the gut as our second brain—a small but agile brain that advises our larger brain about inner and outer threats.[26] There is extensive scientific evidence that reveals the gut impacts our mood, affects our mental and physical health, and even modifies our life choices.[27] Hippocrates was onto something when he said over two thousand years ago that "all disease begins in the gut."

Your gut is chock-full of nerves. In fact, your bowels contain as many nerves as your entire spinal cord, and they relay their signals directly to the brain. If your eyes see someone being injured, or your ears hear a massive percussion blast, your gut feels it. The ancient reptilian brain, sitting beneath the larger cerebral hemispheres that manage consciousness, relays signals straight past the big brain to the site of gut feelings. The result is that we are super sensitive to threats. Literally using our gut as a guide, we can detect threats that we would otherwise miss using our big brain alone.

Over thousands of generations, the small advantage conferred by heightened gut feelings provided a survival benefit. This probably explains why soldiers develop gastrointestinal distress in the midst of extraordinarily stressful combat, or why residents in Nicaragua developed long-standing abdominal pain and diarrhea for decades after the brutality of the Sandinista revolution in the 1980s.[28] Most of us do not face extraordinary physical threats in our immediate environment—no actual combat or lions lurking in wait. Whereas the brain-gut mechanism may have been advantageous ten thousand years ago, it no longer provides the same degree of survival benefit. But gut feelings persist because we still need a visceral alarm system.

This may explain why about 10 percent of the world's population suffers from IBS, which is the most prevalent cause of chronic visceral pain.[29] If you don't have IBS yourself, then you probably know someone who does. Although there are competing explanations for what causes IBS, there is general consensus that it results from an abnormal brain-gut axis.[30]

In his authoritative book, *The Mind-Gut Connection*, my postdoctoral mentor and UCLA professor, Emeran Mayer, explains how IBS is partly a consequence of chronic stress.[31] Elevated stress hormone levels trigger an array of gut changes, including effects on the bacteria lining the intestines, changes in contractions of the bowels, and increased immune activity in the digestive system. These physiologic changes create an emotion that is unique to the gut called visceral anxiety—a special form of anxiety marked by hypervigilance to gut feelings. People with visceral anxiety develop profound emotional responses from hair-trigger gut feelings. They have supercharged little brains that ensure highly sensitive threat detection but that also consign their big brain to a life of anxiety. Even if you fall outside the range of pathologic gut feelings, you probably still experience these sensations. And they may bubble up more often than you'd like.

Next, the interoceptive system detects visceral anxiety and feeds signals to the brain where they register as gut feelings, which is the mental experience of visceral anxiety. These feelings, in turn, lead to cognitions, like believing there is something seriously wrong or deciding to stay near a bathroom at all times or avoiding certain kinds of food that could provoke another bout of visceral anxiety. These cognitions may lead to more stress, even higher levels of stress hormone in the body, and more visceral pain. Over time, this leads to a vicious cycle of worsening visceral anxiety, more gut feelings, and a spiral into maladaptive cognitions and behaviors. It's a cycle that needs to be broken.

Doctors try to break the cycle by addressing downstream events in the gut. Some use antibiotics, probiotics, or specialized diets to alter the gut bacteria. Others use medicines that speed up or slow down gut contractions to blunt the physiologic effects of visceral anxiety. All of these treatments are supported by evidence, although some are more effective than others. But the most effective approach, based on meta-analysis of clinical trials, is to reduce the body's stress response. Treatments like mindful meditation, cognitive behavioral therapy, dynamic psychotherapy, relaxation training, antidepressants, and even hypnotherapy are all supported by randomized controlled trials.[32] If these treatments work to restore a healthy brain-gut axis through stress reduction, then it figures that VR might also work for IBS through the same mechanisms.

After seeing the initial success with the hospitalized IBS patient on ketamine, I decided to perform a larger study to test the effect of VR on visceral pain. My research team evaluated VR in a group of thirty-three hospitalized patients who were experiencing visceral pain from a variety of causes that included IBS, inflammatory bowel disease, pancreatitis, and diverticulitis. We compared their response to VR against another group of hospitalized patients with somatic pain who also used VR. A third group of patients with a combination of pain types did not receive VR at all. We found that VR was better than no VR across all types of pain, that it worked equally well for both visceral and somatic pain, and that it provided an average symptom reduction of around 25 percent.[33] A separate study conducted by University of Cambridge psychologists James Pamment and Jane Aspell found that inducing a virtual out-of-body experience allowed patients with chronic pain, including IBS patients, to reduce their pain by 37 percent after the illusion.[34]

We still need more research to test VR in patients with visceral pain. In the meantime, the studies to date support VR as another effective mind-based treatment for conditions like IBS. Together with a growing number of gastroenterologists around the world, I routinely use VR in my clinic alongside traditional medical therapies. I discuss my experiences with these treatments in Part II. Later, in Part III, I explain how a specialized gut biosensor may help patients rewire their interoceptive signaling through VR-enabled biofeedback therapy.

In this chapter we explored the psychology and neuroscience of how perception, which we can manipulate powerfully with VR, influences our experience of pain. We learned that VR can render pain invisible through inattentional blindness. It is a fast-forward button to speed through episodes of pain. It nips pain signals in the bud by shutting pain gates in the spinal cord. It can insulate the mind from the physical and affective consequences of pain. And finally, it can dampen inner pain of both somatic and visceral origin.

Up to this point, we have explored the role of VR for conditions marked by heightened awareness of events around us and within us. In Chapter 2, we discussed how hypervigilance of external events, like how we're treated by other people or how we respond to frightening triggers, can lead to anxiety. In this chapter we covered how hypervigilance of inner pain signals can lead to physical and emotional suffering. But there are also conditions where people have too little connection with their inner and outer worlds. If VR can loosen up a tight and domineering mind, can it also tighten a loose and disassociated mind?

CHAPTER FOUR

Becoming Whole

Richard Breton is facing his inner demon. Literally. Breton, a fifty-four-year-old man who suffers from uncontrollable hallucinations, is staring at a satanic figure with two ram-like horns, blood-red skin, and massive bat wings.

"You are no good," says the figure in a dark and ominous voice. "You are a bad father. You are a bad husband. You are worthless."

These are tough words to hear. But that's exactly what Breton deals with every day as his own personal Lucifer chides, insults, and distracts him incessantly. He can't shake the demon from his head. His quality of life has paid a price.

Now Breton is confronting his persecutor face-to-face. He is wearing a VR headset that displays a visual depiction of his inner voice. Over the course of seven weekly sessions, Breton enters VR and goes to battle against the intruder, commanding the voice to cease, to leave him in peace, and to find someone else to bother. Breton is not alone in there. He is side by side with his psychiatrist, Alexandre Dumais, who accompanies Breton in the virtual world. But in an unexpected twist, the satanic presence is, in fact, Dumais himself, playing the role of Breton's sinister companion.

"The patient is seeing a concrete representation of his hallucination," explains Dumais, who pioneered this new form of VR-assisted talk therapy at the University of Montreal. "He has a direct dialogue with the hallucination."

The voice talking back comes from Dumais, who is sitting in a nearby room wearing a headset. As he speaks, Dumais's voice is permuted by a computer into devilish tones, piped through the software, and then emerges through the mouth of the virtual avatar.

Breton is the first person to try VR avatar therapy for schizophrenia,[1] a condition that affects around 1 percent of the population across nations, classes, and cultures.[2] At the core of schizophrenia is a fractured sense of self. In contrast to people with anxiety disorders who experience a hypervigilant mind that sets rigid borders between self and other, people with schizophrenia often feel like they cannot stop the world from seeping in. They may hear uncontrollable foreign voices that interrupt without warning. Others may see, smell, or feel things that don't exist. Some become paranoid that other people are eavesdropping on their thoughts. They may feel vulnerable and exposed, as though they have no privacy and are at the whims of their persecutory voices.

The pathogenesis of schizophrenia is complex, but research indicates it occurs, at least in part, from abnormalities in the default mode network of the brain—the self-referential system we discussed in Chapter 2. Whereas the default mode network is hyperactive in conditions like anxiety or depression, neuroimaging reveals that people with schizophrenia have disrupted connections in the same network.[3] Recent evidence indicates that long-term clinical outcomes of schizophrenia are related to the degree of default mode network connectivity; the more disconnected the network, the poorer the outcomes.[4]

The mainstay of treatment for schizophrenia is to use antipsychotic drugs like aripiprazole, risperidone, and clozapine, among others. These drugs work by changing the levels of dopamine and serotonin in the brain, which may help normalize connections within the default mode network.[5] Targeting neurotransmitters can be very effective in reducing hallucinations and may also diminish paranoid delusions, but around 30 percent of people continue to have debilitating symptoms despite pharmacotherapy.[6]

Beyond drug therapy, many people with schizophrenia receive cognitive behavioral therapy, also called CBT, to supplement their medical therapy. With CBT, therapists use talk therapy to help their clients identify and redirect unhelpful and distressing thoughts. The goal is to teach patients how to recognize when a hallucination is occurring and take steps to intervene.

Regrettably, the theory of CBT does not always translate into reality with schizophrenia. Although CBT can help some patients, research shows that its clinical benefit is low to moderate, at best.[7] CBT is limited because it's challenging for therapists to recreate a patient's hallucinations. Without a reliable way of introducing realistic scenarios, therapists are constrained to discussing how best to handle hallucinations once they arise—a theoretical exercise with limited durable impact. Of course, patients may experience active hallucinations in the midst of CBT, but therapists cannot access the phenomena directly.

That's what motivated Dumais to develop a new form of CBT that enables a three-way trialogue between a patient, the patient's inner voices, and the patient's therapist. Before entering VR, Dumais worked with Breton to characterize the inner voice and give it a literal face using the same type of Identi-Kit software police use to profile a wanted criminal. But rather than building the likeness of a scofflaw, Dumais created a faithful reproduction of Breton's inner bully. By toggling switches and pushing buttons on a digital dashboard, Dumais can fine-tune the avatar's facial features, skin color, shape, and size. He can make it grow wings and horns, wear a pair of glasses, or have a beard. He can make the persecutor look like a human, a zombie, a reptile, or a furry animal. There's an infinite number of possible demons lurking in the software; the trick is to pick one that best aligns with each patient's inner world. Then, once the visuals are complete, Dumais modifies his own voice to sound like the unique voice ringing in his patient's ears. After he gets it right through trial and error, Dumais is ready to enter his patient's inner reality through virtual reality.

Once inside, Dumais assumes the avatar's identity and interacts with his patient. With Breton, he pushes back hard at first, parroting sentiments that Breton commonly hears, like "You are worthless," or "You are a bad father." The heckling continues. But every so often, Dumais breaks character and offers some coaching. He instructs Breton to stand up to the voice, to talk to it and reason with it. This is difficult at first. People with schizophrenia often avoid engaging in a meaningful dialogue with their voice, which they often perceive to be an omnipotent and godlike presence. Yet, by seeing and hearing it within the 3-D world of VR, and by literally staring at it, face-to-face, Breton has little choice but to engage. Over time, the avatar becomes less hostile and more understanding. It progressively backs down, becomes less threatening, and cedes power to Breton. By the end of the seven-week treatment period, the avatar has surrendered and become more of a companion than an enemy, saying things like "You're not as bad as I thought," or "I underestimated you."

When Dumais's program works, patients learn that their voice is not an all-knowing, all-powerful entity. They achieve greater self-efficacy, wrestle control from their persecutor, and become more assertive. Fighting and winning the psychic civil war is an empowering victory. The voice is no longer perceived to be an external, uncontrollable invader. Rather, it becomes a part of oneself.

The treatment worked for Breton. "Before, I used to pray," he told me, reflecting on his life prior to the VR treatment. "I still pray. But now, what I learned in VR is that instead of always praying and just hoping he leaves me, now I can confront him head on." Since the therapy, Breton's intruding voice dropped from fifteen times per day to far fewer. "My worst days could be one, two, three times maximum. On many days I don't hear the voice at all," he said.

Breton's story inspired Dumais to study his treatment in a larger group of patients. He turned to the work of an influential British psychiatrist named Julian Leff, a former faculty member of University College London, who in 2013 invented the original avatar therapy for treatment-resistant schizophrenia.[8] Leff had grown frustrated with the limitations of medication and traditional CBT. He had an insight about why patients feel so helpless despite treatment. "I thought, 'That's not surprising,'" said Leff in an interview for *The Lancet Psychiatry*, "because the voices are invisible. So I wondered, what if we could give them a face?"[9] Inexpensive VR technology was not yet widely available in 2013, so Leff rendered his avatars in 2-D and projected them on a TV screen. After a series of pilot trials, Leff worked with his colleague, Professor Tom Craig, to publish a large, randomized controlled trial in 2018 comparing 2-D avatar therapy versus supportive counseling sessions.[10] They found a large difference in favor of avatar therapy. Not only was there a significant reduction in the frequency of hallucinations, but patients found them to be less distressing, shorter in duration, less disruptive, and more benevolent compared to patients who received supportive counseling. The effect was far greater than traditional CBT, suggesting that adding avatars can boost the effectiveness of talk therapy.

Dumais took the next step by adding VR. In a paper also published in 2018, Dumais and his colleagues followed a similar model as the British research team, but this time added the immersive component he tested with Breton.[11] They randomized patients with treatment-resistant schizophrenia to VR avatar therapy versus usual care, where the latter group received antipsychotic medications and non-VR talk therapy. Once again, the effect was dramatic. Three months after starting therapy, patients in the VR group had fewer and less severe hallucinations and improved quality of life compared to the control group. Importantly, the effect was considerably larger than the already impressive benefits of 2-D avatar therapy observed by the British team. To give a sense of the difference, we can compare 2-D and 3-D therapy on a standardized scale called the "effect size," which starts at zero, meaning no effect, and goes up from there. An effect size of 0.2 is considered small, 0.5 is medium, and 0.8 is large.[12] Whereas Craig and Leff documented an effect size of 0.8 using 2-D avatar therapy, Dumais found an effect size of 1.2 using 3-D VR therapy, which is an extremely large statistical effect. In the absence of a head-to-head trial of 2-D versus 3-D treatment, the indirect evidence suggests that VR provides an incremental benefit over viewing avatars on a 2-D screen.

Moreover, Dumais studied his VR therapy in what he called "ultra-resistant" patients who had already failed medications and CBT. "Our results hold great promise," Dumais wrote, "for even the most difficult-to-treat patients with schizophrenia."[13]

Dumais believes that VR's unique features contribute to its powerful effects for ultra-resistant schizophrenia. By leveraging the technology's flexibility, reproducibility, and ability to enable patients to rehearse new skills in carefully engineered environments, Dumais is offering a new therapy to complement drugs and traditional CBT. In Chapter 2 we saw how these features of VR can help patients with anxiety or depression achieve a psychedelic-like flow state. Here, Dumais leverages the same technology to counteract a fluid state of mind, and instead replace it with a more structured, self-affirming state of control. "VR therapy might alleviate patients' distress by attenuating the threats to the self," he concludes.[14]

Treating schizophrenia requires more than controlling hallucinations. Hallucinations are categorized as positive symptoms by mental health practitioners, meaning there is an excess of normal function (like hearing or seeing things that are not real). But that's only half the problem. There are also negative symptoms of schizophrenia, meaning a reduction or loss of normal function. Negative symptoms include blunted emotions, low motivation, or little interest in social engagement. Therapists not only need to quash the positive symptoms but also counteract the negative symptoms.

Social isolation is among the most treatment-resistant negative symptoms of schizophrenia. Antipsychotics are largely ineffective for managing social impairment, and CBT offers only modest benefits. But there is evidence that social skills training, also called SST, can help.[15] With SST, therapists teach patients how to scan for social cues and respond appropriately. For example, many people with schizophrenia have trouble looking other people in the eyes or have difficulty noticing facial expressions, often because they falsely believe people are staring back judgmentally. SST teaches patients how to overcome their misleading cognitions, proactively interpret body language, and make positive social connections. Still, it's hard to practice SST in real-life scenarios, plus the availability of skilled therapists is limited. VR can help here, too.

A team of psychologists at Vanderbilt University led by Sohee Park and Laura Adery created a VR program that recreates common social settings.[16] They surround their patients in busy public spaces, like a market or restaurant, and send them on missions to accomplish tasks they would otherwise avoid. In one simulation, patients are challenged to strike up a conversation with someone waiting at a bus stop and find out their favorite TV show. In another, they're instructed to join a table occupied by strangers in a crowded cafeteria. Not easy stuff. Speaking for myself, even contemplating these tasks rekindles memories of pimply faced high school angst; I can only imagine how someone with paranoid schizophrenia approaches these difficult encounters.

But the program goes a step further. To up the challenge, Park and Adery fill their environment with avatars that can appear either friendly or downright mean, depending on how they're programmed. The researchers dial up the intensity as patients become more comfortable in the virtual environment. People begin to turn and stare unblinkingly. Families stop what they're doing and look over, as if judging the patient for just being in their midst. It's very unpleasant, yet the patients still try to carry out their missions despite the creepy stares.

Patients are not abandoned in these socially awkward environments. Just like in Dumais's virtual world, therapists in Park and Adery's world are nearby to coach patients throughout the scenes. If an avatar looks unpleasant, for example, the therapist might ask the patient to come up with a reason for the unpleasant reaction other than a personal judgment. Patients learn to recognize they might not be the subject of scorn or personal indictment, and that other people have their own inner lives that can be misinterpreted. Through trial and error, the software allows patients to rehearse social interactions and try out different dialogues and techniques. In the process, they gain a sense of self-empowerment over

their negative symptoms, just like Dumais's software offers empower-
ment over the positive symptoms.

The Vanderbilt team studied their virtual SST program in a clinical trial. Patients with schizophrenia completed ten VR treatments, each
thirty minutes in length, over the course of a five-week study period. The
results were dramatic. Ninety-four percent of the participants rated the
program as enjoyable. Although it was challenging for many patients to
work through the social missions, most were able to persist and come
away feeling better equipped for social engagements. Negative symptoms improved across the board, with both statistically significant and
clinically important benefits. The clinical effect size of VR therapy was
medium to large in caliber, which is impressive given how hard it is to
mitigate social impairment with usual treatments.

"It has given me a new set of proper social skills to use," said one
participant. "It has enlightened me so much. I had no idea that my social
skills were a little off and this research has given me a new hold on it."

"I use the skills in the tests and apply them to real life," said another
participant, emphasizing the durability of the treatment. "I learned how
to be a better listener."[17]

These testimonials reveal that immersion can make a difference in
the lives of people with schizophrenia in a way that medication cannot.
But beyond personal anecdotes, the scientific evidence is growing every
year. A literature review conducted by Mar Rus-Calafell of King's College London found another *fifty* studies testing VR for psychosis, and
that review was published in 2018, meaning there's even more evidence
now.[18] After steeping herself in the research, Rus-Calafell concluded that
it's time to put VR into the hands of more doctors and patients. "This is
definitely something we have to do—we must," she told the trade publication *Psychiatry Advisor*. "It's evidence-based and can make our lives
easier. You can offer treatment as much as you want so you can repeat the
exposure; because you've got it there, you don't have the excuse of saying
'I cannot go out with my patient to try these out.' You have it in your
clinical setting."[19]

This core idea—that VR allows clinicians to go beyond the couch—
is opening new ways to expand the patient-provider relationship. For

conditions marked by an eroded sense of self, where the limits of traditional talk therapy make it challenging to access a patient's inner world, VR offers a gateway into a fractured mind and an opportunity to rebuild its parts from within.

Next, let's see how VR can help with another condition of disrupted identity that affects nearly fifty million people worldwide.

Just outside the Dutch capital of Amsterdam lies a small village called Hogeweyk that is like no other community in the world. The village is surrounded by a wall and has only one entrance that is carefully monitored twenty-four hours a day. Nobody enters or exits without clearance. Inside the wall are 152 residents who have one thing in common: every one of them has advanced dementia. The citizens of this unique community are all living with a fractured identity. Hogeweyk was created to restore their sense of self.

Dementia is not a disease unto itself but a group of symptoms caused by other diseases, most commonly Alzheimer's disease and stroke. In other words, very different conditions create similar deficits in thinking and memory. The most common cause of dementia is Alzheimer's, a neurodegenerative disease in which a protein called beta-amyloid forms plaques throughout the brain. These plaques disrupt normal brain function and cause progressive cognitive decline.

Although Alzheimer's disease and schizophrenia are clinically dissimilar and affect different age groups, they share a common feature: both exhibit disconnects within the default mode network.

"If you look at Alzheimer's disease and you look at whether it attacks a particular part of the brain," says Marcus Raichle, the neuroscientist noted in Chapter 2 who famously described our default mode of thinking, "what's amazing is that it actually attacks the default mode network."[20]

Just like with schizophrenia, where the default mode network disintegrates and leaves behind a disrupted sense of self, patients with Alzheimer's also suffer from a disintegrated self. Neuroimaging reveals that the default mode network disconnects in a very specific way in Alzheimer's disease, right between an area called the posterior cingulate cortex, which supports awareness, and the hippocampus, which governs memory.[21] This detachment causes a profound breakdown in identity. Because the hippocampus is cut loose from the rest of the network, patients can no longer form short-term memories, and they become unable to transcribe a personal narrative. It's as though an inner tape recorder stops working, and then everything after that point is struck from the record. But in the case of Alzheimer's dementia, there is still a way to access and restore the archived recordings from before the malfunction, and that offers some hope for treatment.

Research shows that people with Alzheimer's can reconstitute aspects of their lost identity if they are reminded of memories that predate the dementia.[22] This is because the brain is "plastic," a term used by neuroscientists to describe the brain's ability to reshape in response to new demands. Our central nervous system is not like a stagnant block of Play-Doh; rather, it is a living, breathing, shape-shifting part of our body, and its structure and function can change over time. When the human brain is placed in an enriching environment it can rewire its circuitry to strengthen existing connections and reform broken links. In the field of stroke rehabilitation, cognitive and physical training help expedite the brain's recovery, often allowing new circuits to form in and around damaged areas. The same is true for people with dementia: surrounding these people with memories of a forgotten past can enhance thinking and rehabilitate memory. But when they are not offered a means of self-rediscovery, patients with dementia face relentless cognitive decline, severe depression, and social isolation.

These findings led geriatricians to develop a treatment called reminiscence therapy in which they rekindle memories in their patients using photographs, nostalgic personal items, or familiar music from a bygone era. In a typical program, patients regularly meet with a therapist, often in partnership with family caregivers, and relive their personal stories with the aid of memory tools. Clinical trials reveal that reminiscence therapy can improve cognitive abilities, enhance mood, prevent unintended wandering, and calm aggression in people with dementia by tapping into the brain's plasticity.

This brings us back to Hogeweyk. The community architects studied reminiscence therapy and decided to build an environment that leverages the brain's capacity for change. If patients with dementia could be surrounded by an enriching environment, 24/7, then maybe they could rediscover their identity and, at the very least, experience a slowdown in cognitive decline. In lieu of a traditional nursing home, where patients are often confined to sterile and uncreative spaces, Hogeweyk features homes built to resemble specific eras like the 1950s, 1970s, and 2000s. Residents are assigned to live in a house that most closely matches the time predating their dementia. Everything from the furnishings to the tablecloths to the wall decorations are carefully selected to reflect a period that feels familiar and comforting to the residents.

The citizens of Hogeweyk are encouraged to leave their homes and explore the surrounding village, which includes a post office, grocery store, hair salon, and other shops tastefully arranged around a central town square. Like a real-life version of *The Truman Show*, where Jim Carrey's character lives within a fabricated town as the star of a reality TV show, the residents of Hogeweyk meander about their village while surveyed by a team of 250 employees hired to safeguard their security and well-being. But unlike the Hollywood movie, the goal of Hogeweyk is to cocoon its residents in a brain-boosting environment that's custom-built to slow the ravages of dementia through reminiscence therapy and high-touch care.

The results of Hogeweyk have been nothing short of remarkable. Compared to residents with dementia at traditional senior care facilities, the citizens of Hogeweyk show signs of improved cognitive function, enhanced quality of life, less depression, better nutrition, and a longer lifespan. Although a head-to-head clinical trial has not been performed, the results speak for themselves, says Yvonne van Amerongen, founder and director of Hogeweyk. In an interview with CNN's Dr. Sanjay Gupta, she laid out the facts: "We see that people are invited to exercise more because everyone can go outside and walk in the sun. We see that people meet others here. This life helps people to get strong. We haven't had scientific research on living longer, but in 1992 when we started this, people came in with the same indication, and they would stay an average of two-and-a-half years. Now they live three-and-a-half years. It's not scientific. But I can count."[23]

Based on the success of Hogeweyk, other communities are beginning to rethink the role of nursing homes and long-term care facilities. In 2018, a similar village called Glenner Town Square opened in San Diego. It is replete with a city hall, museum, library, and a Disney-like Main Street featuring a 1959 Ford Thunderbird parked in front of a diner.[24] The designers even hired a Hollywood prop company to provide historically accurate furniture and install rubberized props, like fire hydrants and retro street signs. Other "dementia villages," as they're now called, are planned for over one hundred cities across the United States and beyond.

Hogeweyk pioneered a new way of engaging seniors that is being replicated across the globe. But with a massive and still growing population of nearly fifty million people with dementia, we need a lot more Hogeweyks to keep up. How can we scale the benefits of reminiscence therapy with so few sites available to meet the burgeoning needs of the aging population?

In Brookdale Quincy Bay, a senior living community in Quincy, Massachusetts, ten residents gather in an unassuming fluorescent-lit meeting room for a group therapy session. But unlike their usual meetings, this time each participant is wearing a VR headset. All the headsets are directly controlled by Reed Hayes, an MIT graduate student who sits among the seniors with a tablet computer in his lap, ready to dial up a virtual field trip. The first destination is the French countryside.

"Ohhhh!" they all say in unison.

"It's unbelievable!" says one. "Oh my god!" says another.

Next, they travel together to the depths of the ocean.

"Oh, look at that fish!"

The group is abuzz. They're talking, laughing, and utterly amazed at what they're seeing. There is a palpable energy in the room. These seniors have left the four walls of their nursing home on a fantastic voyage.

Then, after touring Venice, Italy, and visiting the Yosemite Valley, everyone arrives at the front yard of a modest single-story home. The house is unfamiliar to all but one resident, Maryanne, whose virtual journey has just left her dumbfounded.

"You recognize the house?" asks Hayes from behind his computer. Everyone is silent except Maryanne.

"Yeah, well, wait a minute," she says, trying to sort out what she's seeing. "Oh, don't say that," she says, jaw agape. She places both hands over her mouth in astonishment. "Well, that's the most beautiful place in the world! *Who did this?*"

Maryanne is now back at the home she shared for years with her husband. She cannot believe what she's seeing. At a loss for words, she begins to sob uncontrollably. The others are silent, just taking in the moment. They have traveled with Maryanne to revisit part of her forgotten past. They are no longer in their senior living community. Now they are together with Maryanne at her former home, which is digitally reconstructed in 360-degree images, thanks to a VR version of Google Earth. Her companions are right beside her as she confronts a flood of powerful memories. She is speechless. Her companions break into a round of supportive applause. Everyone laughs together as Maryanne cries tears of joy.[25]

"It was a spark," says Hayes, the Wizard of Oz behind the headsets. "Without the VR she didn't remember the house. She didn't remember that her husband used to work at the back of the house, or that she raised her children there. It all came back in VR."

After witnessing the power of VR for people like Maryanne, Hayes cofounded a startup company called Rendever that focuses on VR for senior care. "We noticed that once they were done with the demo they'd go back to their friends and talk about what they experienced. It was social. Can you imagine coming up with a new conversation after being there ten years and you haven't been out?"[26]

Kyle Rand, the current CEO of Rendever, cofounded the company with Hayes. A Duke graduate who studied neuroscience, Rand started Rendever after watching his grandmother struggle with social isolation in her senior living community. It struck him that VR could recreate the magic of Hogeweyk, but without needing the resources and space required to build an entire dementia village.

Until thousands more Hogeweyks are spread across the globe, there will be an unmet need to engage seniors within the confines of traditional care communities. As innovative as it is, even Hogeweyk is limited in space and resources. VR is different, because it can deliver infinitely more environments than any brick-and-mortar facility.

Rand thinks we can do more with existing senior communities, which he believes often fall short in serving their residents. "These are organizations built around the idea of community, and people pay a lot of money for their loved ones to get into them," Rand told me. "And then they sit around watching TV and not engaging with the world. It's sad and also dangerous. If you spend years watching TV and doing little outside of that it's inevitable there will be some cognitive decline."

Rand is careful to explain that he's not trying to cure dementia. "We're just finding a way for people to become more connected to the world, more connected to each other, and more connected to themselves," he said. "VR is a platform that can help seed conversations and bring people out of their shells."[27]

Rand's company offers a library of curated VR worlds for senior centers. In one program, called *Balloon Poppers*, a group travels to a calming beach with colored balloons floating in the air. Each player is instructed to pop all the balloons of a specific color. Whoever pops all their assigned balloons first wins the game. "It's like digital bingo," says Rand. "Seniors love competition. Interactive games cultivate positive group play and engagement."

In the United Kingdom, a team of developers is also using VR to address dementia by recreating indelible moments from history. Scott Gorman and Arfa Rehman built a VR library called LookBack that delivers what they call "immersive reminiscent experiences" customized for people with dementia. In one experience, for example, Gorman and Rehman filmed a 360-degree reenactment of a woman buying goods in a drugstore to prepare for Queen Elizabeth II's 1953 coronation, which for many British elders was a magical moment. In another LookBack experience, seniors travel to a 1960s version of Brighton beach in the UK, where sunbathers wear vintage swimsuits and bathing caps.

Like Kyle Rand, Gorman had family members in senior communities that he found suboptimal. "They were far from the kinds I wanted to be able to afford," Gorman told *The Daily Beast* in an interview. "They didn't have the luxury of a precreated village. In fact they were pretty sterile, and not stimulating at all. So I think people are very curious and eager for inexpensive solutions that can improve quality of life."[28]

The anecdotes are powerful, but is there scientific evidence to support VR reminiscence therapy? In 2017, an MIT graduate student named Charles Lin put the Rendever system to the test as the subject of his dissertation.[29] He studied sixty-three people among four assisted living communities. Two of the sites were assigned the VR intervention, and the others were assigned to watching TV. In both cases, participants used their assigned technology for twenty minutes each day over the course of two weeks. Lin found that by the end of the study, residents assigned to VR had lower anxiety and depression scores, increased ability to perform vigorous activity, and higher perception of overall health compared to the control group. The VR group also expressed higher levels of "trust" for other residents and staff compared to those who watched TV, emphasizing the positive impact of VR on social function and mimicking the effect of VR in Park and Adery's schizophrenia social isolation research.

Beyond virtual reminiscence therapy, the literature is now full of studies demonstrating other benefits of VR for dementia care. In one randomized trial from Chang Gung University in Taiwan, for example, patients who learned tai chi exercises in a VR headset showed meaningful improvements in cognitive and physical function compared to a non-VR control (effect sizes of 0.5 to 0.8).[30] At the University of Southern California, neuroscientist Judy Pa created a game called *Neurorider* in which patients pedal a stationary bicycle and navigate through a virtual park.[31] The program is designed to enhance memory function in the hippocampus, that part of the default mode network taken off-line in Alzheimer's. Scientists at the University of Milan are also using stationary bikes, but allowing seniors to ride together in groups from the comfort of their homes using a game called *SocialBike*.[32] A research team in Greece created a virtual supermarket with shopping tasks that is over 90 percent accurate at detecting the earliest signs of cognitive impairment in people at risk for dementia.[33] At UCLA, neuroscientist Nanthia Suthana combined VR with a surgically implanted prosthesis to learn how people with dementia create new memories as they navigate a 3-D environment.[34] And in perhaps the most ambitious global study yet, the Alzheimer's Research UK foundation created a VR game called *Sea Hero Quest* that tests spatial navigation.[35] Over four million people from nearly every country have played the game and donated their results to science. The researchers are using the crowd-sourced data to set global benchmarks for how well people can navigate in 3-D space, and they are applying these normed results to identify people with the earliest signs of Alzheimer's.

Together with the schizophrenia research, these worldwide examples in dementia care reveal the potential of VR to address two of humanity's most intractable mental health conditions. VR cannot remove the amyloid plaques of Alzheimer's disease or awaken every cognitively impaired senior from the moribund depths of bewilderment. But for some people, sometimes, VR can restore a sense of awe. It can enable patients and their providers to visit therapeutic wonderlands. It can offer a powerful technique to reconnect people to the world around them. And perhaps most important, it can open new windows upon the mind, allowing people with a fractured identity to rediscover who they are, if only in glimpses.

CHAPTER FIVE

Mind the Gap

THE JET ENGINES HAVE JUST FIRED UP AND LOGAN IS GETTING NERvous. A twenty-five-year-old jujitsu master, Logan can take a punch. But not when he's on an airplane. There's something about being in a fuselage that robs his courage and weakens his strength. Now his heart is racing, his skin is slick with sweat, and his pupils are dilating as he looks out the window of a Qantas Airbus A330 that's about to leave his hometown of Sydney, Australia.

The plane begins to accelerate. Logan's seat vibrates as the engines reach full power. The wheels bump over the seams in the tarmac, at first slowly, then faster, and faster still, as the plane achieves takeoff velocity. He hears the overhead compartment rattling and wonders if it's about to spring open and release its cargo. Logan is white-knuckling his seat and is rigid with fear. He looks away from the window and rests his gaze on the passenger next to him, trying to distract his mind from the sensory onslaught. But he is gripped with terror. He's convinced it was a huge risk to board this plane. Only luck will get him off alive.

But it is too late. The plane lifts off. Logan peers out the window and watches the runway fade into the distance. The terminal buildings now look like small boxes. And here come the clouds. His chair rumbles as low-level turbulence rocks the plane. The wing outside his window is flapping and bending; it seems too massive to sustain the pressure. Logan's gasping for air and panicked. He can't take it for another minute.

"Okay, okay," says Les Posen, Logan's clinical psychologist. "You can remove the headset now."

Logan never left the ground. He experienced a VR simulation of his worst fear. He sat in a real airline seat from an Airbus A330 that quite literally shook his body. And the jet engine sounds were booming from specialized bass-enhanced speakers. But what he saw came through a headset. Everything Logan experienced, from the bone-rattling turbulence to the bouncing wing, was an elaborate setup in Les Posen's office in Melbourne, Australia.

Logan has struggled with flight phobia for most of his life. He is so afraid of airplanes that he decided to drive—not fly—the 550-mile journey from Sydney to Melbourne to visit Posen, who is among the world's leading experts on VR phobia therapy. Ironically, Logan's car trip culminated in a series of VR airplane flights.

"Let's try that again," says Posen. "But this time I'm going to wire you up and measure your stress." Posen clips a sensor over Logan's right index finger. The sensor connects to a nearby computer, and a dashboard lights up on the screen and reveals a slow, undulating line. Posen instructs Logan to wear the headset again. Now Logan is back in the plane and poised for takeoff. Posen monitors the signal closely.

"Interesting," he observes. "You're in the green zone right now. That's unexpected."

By "green zone," Posen means that Logan is not yet showing physical signs of stress. The sensor is measuring Logan's heart rate, but it's doing much more than that. Unto itself, heart rate cannot really tell what's going on in someone's mind and body. A racing heart could imply terror, or it could just mean excitement; there's a big difference. Posen is looking for something more subtle and telling. He's studying the beat-to-beat variation in heart rate as Logan prepares for takeoff.

This metric, called heart rate variability, or HRV, informs Posen about what's happening between Logan's mind and body. Recall from Chapter 3 that the brain and gut are connected by the vagus nerve, the equivalent of a high-speed network cable that sends messages back and forth. It turns out the vagus nerve also connects the brain to the heart, not just to the gut. When people are relaxed or highly focused, the vagus not only signals the heart to slow down but also conditions the heart to be more responsive to breathing. In a state of calm, the heart slows down a tiny bit on each exhale and speeds up a touch on each inhale. That's healthy. But in times of stress, the vagus nerve becomes overwhelmed and the heart both speeds up *and* loses its rhythmic connection with breathing.

But for Logan, despite sitting in a plane at the end of the runway, his heart is still synced to his breath, indicating a state of relative calm. The HRV sensor shows him in the green zone, meaning that even though his heart may be speeding up a bit, the terror is still in check.

"I thought you'd at least be in the blue zone by now, if not the red zone," says Posen.

"But I feel stressed just sitting here," Logan responds.

"You may *feel* stressed, but your body isn't showing the stress yet. There's a disconnect between your mind and your body."

This is a critical insight. Somehow, Logan's mental self is not synced with his corporeal self. He feels fear even before his body begins to sweat, pant, or tremble. Psychologists call this anticipation anxiety. It's as though Logan's overthinking mind is preparing for the inevitable. He's jumping the gun. Posen has a theory.

"You practice jujitsu, right?" he asks.

"Yeah. But it doesn't seem to help me on a plane."

"Don't be so sure of that," Posen says. "Do you practice breathing exercises in jujitsu?"

"All the time. It's a big part of jujitsu. I'm always aware of my breath."

Posen connects the dots.

"That's why you're still in the green zone right now. You don't know it yet, but you're able to control your fear at this point from all your training. Your heart is still beating in sync with your lungs. Your body is still in control, even if your mind thinks otherwise. You are still in command. Let's see what happens next."

Posen toggles some switches on his computer. The jet engines fire up again. The seat vibrates. The airplane rolls down the runway. Posen monitors the HRV data as Logan grips his seat and tenses his body.

"There you go," says Posen. "You went right through the green zone into the red zone."

Logan is panicking again. His chest is heaving and his skin is sweaty.

"What are you feeling?"

"Scared."

"No, I mean literally. What are you feeling inside of your body?"

Logan stops for a second to think.

"I feel tense inside. I feel my heart beating out of my chest. I feel my lungs straining. I feel my hands gripping."

"Good. Now *this* is fear. What you felt before was not yet fear. It was a false alarm. I want you to remember what you're feeling now," says Posen, "because *this* is your body in fear."

Like many people with phobias, Logan's brain does not always sync with his body. Even when his body remains calm and unperturbed, as it was at the beginning of the flight simulation, his mind still assumes the worst. It's as though his mind refuses to accept that his body is okay. Worse still, Logan's brain sends signals that trigger a strong emotional response in his body, setting off a vicious cycle of panic. The key for successful treatment, according to Posen, is for Logan to interpret his body signals more effectively before things get out of hand. He needs to bridge the divide between brain and body. VR can help mind the gap.

Posen uses VR to recreate emotional triggers with fidelity, expose his patients to their worst fear, and then help them monitor their body's response. "If you can't measure it, you can't manage it," Posen says. "The HRV sensor is like an emotion barometer. I use it to guide my patients and show them—literally show them—what's happening in their body."

By measuring HRV, Posen offers his patients a way to see and feel what they might otherwise struggle to detect. For Logan, visualizing his mind-body dialogue allows him to modulate his emotions and cognitions using VR-enabled biofeedback. Ultimately, he'll also learn to alter his behaviors, which are inadvertently reinforcing his fear response.

We can understand how this works by again applying the theory of embodied cognitions that was discussed in Chapter 1. Here, Posen uses VR to convince Logan he's on an airplane by tweaking his senses through visual, tactile, and auditory stimulation. This fools his body into assuming a first-person perspective in the seat of an Airbus A330 readying for takeoff. At first, Logan's body remains steady and calm, indicating a window of opportunity to maintain control before his strong emotions take over. But as the simulation continues, his heart races, his skin moistens, and his muscles tighten. These events trigger the interoceptive system—that army of inner sentinels standing guard to inform central command of trouble—to warn the brain with urgent messages. Logan is overwhelmed by a feeling of imminent demise. This feeling reinforces his cognition that air travel is an existential hazard that must be avoided at all costs.

Because Logan so quickly misreads his inner signals as evidence of physical danger, he doesn't normally have a chance to interrupt the inexorable cycle of panic. But with the HRV sensor, Logan can better align his mind with the physiologic reality of his body. As he becomes more skilled at reading his body, he gets better at staving off his emotional response, tamping down his feelings, and most important, forming a new cognition that flying is not a life-or-death decision.

Posen dials up the VR intensity in a controlled and gradual manner as the training progresses, pushing Logan's mind and body just past their previous set point. For Logan, this graded exposure is like being in a digital dojo, where he can repeatedly practice mind-body focus in exactly the setting he needs the most. After just a few sessions, Logan is able to stay in the green zone for the entire takeoff.

Adam Gazzaley, the neuroscientist we discussed in Chapter 2 and met in Chapter 3, has taken Posen's setup to the next level. Gazzaley created what he calls the "sensory immersion vessel," an enclosed oblong chamber with gull-wing doors, a sporty exterior, and a luxurious interior. From the outside, it looks like a Tesla vehicle, and it's wired to engage mind and body in ways never before realized.[1]

"Think of a sensory deprivation tank," Gazzaley explained to me, "and imagine its exact opposite. That's the sensory immersion vessel. It surrounds our ancient brain in a vibrant high-tech world."

Climb inside and you'll find a multisensory biofeedback experience designed to synchronize mind and body. The interior features a VR headset with the highest resolution imaging currently available. There's a surround-sound system with spatial acoustics, meaning sound comes from all directions in sync with the visuals. The vessel is preloaded with hundreds of scents to recreate the olfactory experience of diverse environments (think cedarwood in a forest, or ocean mist on the beach). The chamber can heat up or cool off, as needed, and it can direct wind to the head, body, or feet. The floor has vibration motors that trigger the sense of touch, and there's even a blanket embedded with sensors to detect and transmit motion on the front of the body. Gazzaley's chamber is a reminder that immersion can go far beyond a headset. Even though vision is a powerful therapeutic stimulus if used wisely, manipulating all the senses offers even more capacity to achieve positive outcomes.

As people settle in, the vessel begins to track a range of biodata. It monitors eye position to detect attention, tracks limb position to measure physical activity, and measures heart rate, HRV, respiratory rate, and even beads of sweat on the skin to estimate levels of stress and arousal. "This is about deep immersion," Gazzaley explains. "It's about harmonizing mind and body by tightly synchronizing all the senses and achieving the unity effect."

When Gazzaley speaks of the unity effect, he is referring to a neuroscience principle that when multiple senses are stimulated at the exact same time, the observer perceives them to represent a single event rather than separate events. For example, if you see someone's mouth moving and simultaneously hear a voice from the same direction, you naturally assume the sight and the sound are related. But if there is a disconnect between senses, like with a badly overdubbed foreign movie translation, the brain has trouble integrating the mismatched stimuli. "The idea is that if I can stimulate all your senses in perfect unison in, say, a beautiful nature scene," Gazzaley continues, "then this synchronized experience can displace other burdens of mind and unlock new perceptions for restoration and transformation."

This description sounds a lot like the flow states we explored in Chapter 2, but here Gazzaley adds a layer of biofeedback to keep mind and body in sync. His immersion vessel employs what neurophysiologists call a closed-loop system. In a closed loop, the brain is first exposed to a stimulus that triggers a response in the body. Next, the inner body signals are measured with sensors. Finally, the sensors transform their data into new stimuli that feed directly back into the brain, completing the brain-body cycle.[2]

In the case of Gazzaley's immersion vessel, the sensory inputs trick the brain into believing it's on a beach or in a forest, or wherever Gazzaley wants it to be. The more senses that are nudged, and the more synchronously they're nudged, the deeper the sense of immersion in the virtual environment. This triggers body reactions that form a positive emotion, like goosebumps, tingling on the skin, a drop in stress hormone levels, slowed breathing, and increased HRV. An array of body sensors records these signals. Rather than verbally describing the sensor results, as Posen does with his HRV data, Gazzaley uses these body signals to update the environment within the vessel, providing an opportunity for biofeedback and even deeper immersion through multisensory integration. For example, as breathing slows down and HRV rises, the scent of cedarwood might become stronger, or the sound of songbirds might become more prominent. These sensory enhancements trigger the brain to pass along even more positive messages to the body, closing the loop.

"The physiologic recordings offer us a comprehensive view of your inner state," Gazzaley explains. "Then we use those recordings to drive the immersion even deeper, engaging the outer senses, and then, again, driving the inner body states." The result is a virtuous cycle of mind-body connectedness, in the literal sense—not in some New Age sense. Gazzaley directly measures the body signals and transmits them straight to the brain, bypassing the interoceptive system altogether. This shortcut is ideal for people like Logan who experience occasional disconnects between mind and body. By translating interoceptive signals into exteroceptive experiences, Gazzaley converts the body's physiology into a metaphorical narrative that is easily accessible to the mind's eye.

Research is bearing out Gazzaley and Posen's vision. In a study led by Alessandra Gorini at the University of Milan, patients with generalized anxiety disorder used VR to explore a tropical island while listening to a relaxation narrative and wearing body sensors that measured skin moisture and heart rate.[3] As the heart rate slowed and sweat dissipated, the sensors triggered peaceful changes in the scenery. Compared to a control group, patients in the VR treatment not only had less anxiety but also curbed their physiologic responses to stress. In another study by Jeff Tarrant of the NeuroMeditation Institute in Oregon, researchers employed brain signals to change the scenery in a virtual environment.[4] Using thoughts alone, patients with anxiety could bring a dying tree back to life or brighten a dimming sun or teleport their body up a waterfall. With repeated practice and training that rewarded positive thinking, patients learned how to flip their brain waves into a calm and restful pattern. Tarrant found that his VR program conferred significant benefits and led to objective changes in brain signaling.

The science of VR biofeedback has resulted in a growing menu of consumer products. Posen uses a system called Psious that is now available to therapists around the world for VR phobia treatment. Gazzaley's new company, Sensync, is marketing his sensory immersion vessel. As of this writing, the only available unit resides at the Four Seasons Hotel in Oahu, Hawaii. Tarrant's VR program is available through a company called Healium that sells a self-branded "biometrically controlled, drugless solution for stress." In Chapter 7, we explore how VR biofeedback not only helps anxiety but also battles chronic pain and reliance on addictive medicines.

Returning to Logan, prior to VR therapy his body would send messages that everything is okay, but his mind ignored the signals and assumed the worst. VR helped him overcome the communication barrier. But for many people the reverse is true: the body advises of trouble, but the mind doesn't get the message and assumes everything is fine. Next, let's see how VR can amplify the body's distress signals and alert the mind when things aren't right.

We all feel sensations on the surface of our body, but how well can you feel sensations *within* your body? It turns out that some people are better than others at focusing within. Here's an exercise to test your ability: using only your inner body sensations, silently count the number of times your heart beats over the next thirty seconds. That's it. Just put down this book, close your eyes if helpful, and count your heartbeats by monitoring your inner body signals. Don't put your hand over your heart, or place your finger on your pulse. Just feel your body from within. Give it a quick try.

How did you do? Was it easy? Or did you struggle to feel one beat from the next? Maybe you focused on your chest. Or perhaps you felt your head bobbing in sync with your heart. Maybe you felt the pulse in your temples, or in your abdomen. For some of you this was difficult. You might have scanned up and down your body seeking a signal but still couldn't detect a solid beat. For others, it might have been pretty easy. Maybe you're one of those people who can sense your body without giving it much thought.

Now ask yourself, on a scale from zero to one hundred, where zero is "not confident at all" and one hundred is "fully confident," how confident are you that you accurately counted the number of heartbeats? Give yourself a score.

You've just performed two tasks that experimental psychologists use to measure the strength of mind-body connection.[5] The first one, called interoceptive accuracy, compares estimated heart rate against actual heart rate. Most people tend to underestimate their actual heart rate when relying only on body signals because it's hard to feel every beat. Interoceptive accuracy is around 66 percent, on average, meaning that two-thirds of heartbeats are accurately detected. The second exercise, called interoceptive awareness, measures confidence in the ability to sense body signals. Some people might be objectively inaccurate but still believe they're highly accurate, indicating not only a physical disconnect between mind and body, but also a cognitive disconnect; they don't know what they don't know. Others are highly accurate and know it. People vary widely along these measures of interoceptive ability.

Research shows that if you're good at monitoring your inner body signals, then you probably experience the world differently from those who are less attuned.[6] This makes sense if we again think of the embodied cognition theory from Chapter 1. When the body experiences strong physical effects from emotions, people who readily detect those effects are more likely to register them intensely compared to those with dampened interoception. Same thing with pain. When the body experiences noxious stimuli, people with high interoception are more likely to feel the pain and suffer its consequences. But when interoception is hindered, people become disconnected from what's happening inside their body. That might be beneficial up to a point because diminished interoception can protect the mind against overwhelming emotions or bolster against pain, but diminished interoception is not beneficial if the mind altogether misses vital messages.

Consider Diana, a twenty-five-year-old graduate student from Milan, Italy, who lost weight precipitously after a stressful period at school.[7] She began to experience intrusive thoughts about being overweight and decided to severely restrict her diet. She monitored her calorie intake obsessively and routinely checked herself in the mirror. Diana was convinced her body was distorted and oversized, so she kept losing weight at an alarming rate of nearly ten pounds per month. It didn't help. She would stare in the mirror crying, still certain of her obesity, even as she became thin as a rail.

Diana began to self-induce vomiting so she could lose even more weight. She grew weak and depressed. Her life was falling apart. Diana's doctors grew concerned and decided to enroll her in an eating disorders clinic at the University of Milan for urgent treatment. Something had to be done.

When Diana checked in she was greeted by a multidisciplinary team that included Giuseppe Riva, a world-renowned psychologist who specializes in immersive therapeutics. Riva had developed a theory that eating disorders like anorexia nervosa—the condition plaguing Diana—partly result from diminished interoception. If the mind cannot tell when the body is wasting away, then patients like Diana might fail to act before it's too late.

Riva decided to measure the strength of Diana's mind-body connection. First, he measured interoceptive accuracy by comparing her estimated heart rate against the real heart rate measured by an electrocardiogram. Diana wasn't even close. In fact, she scored about as low as possible on the test; her estimated heart rate was only 8 percent of the actual heart rate, indicating a near total interoceptive disconnect between mind and body.

Next, Riva measured Diana's interoceptive awareness by asking how confident she was in her estimate. Despite bottoming out on the test, Diana awarded herself a score of ninety-four out of one hundred points for perceived accuracy. She was nearly certain of her estimate. This was a troubling combination: despite being way off in accurately reading her body signals, Diana nonetheless felt like a mind-body guru fully capable of monitoring her inner state.

"Diana's ability to correctly perceive her inner body sensations was severely compromised," Riva explained in a published review of Diana's case. "Nevertheless, she was—at the same time—deeply convinced that her distorted perceptions were correct, thus suggesting a profound detachment between Diana's ability to perceive her body and the awareness of her deficits."[8] Riva believed this mind-body disconnect was a root cause of Diana's illness.

Anorexia nervosa affects about 1 percent of the population and presents with severely restricted food intake, intense fear of gaining weight, and a disturbance in how body weight or shape is experienced. People with anorexia nervosa typically deny the seriousness of low body weight; it's as though their mind is not listening to their body's cry for help. Scientists like Riva, and many others, theorize that anorexia results from a multisensory integration deficit, meaning that patients cannot square their interoceptive signals with beliefs they hold about their body.[9] For example, Diana was certain her body was overweight, so it didn't matter what signals her body sent to the contrary; her mind simply wouldn't accept them. Diana was "locked to a negative body representation," Riva explains, and that perception did not change despite her following a restrictive diet, losing weight, and suffering physical consequences. Her mind ignored her body.

We all have a sense of what Riva calls our internal reality. We literally feel that internal reality through interoception. Over time, through the process of forming embodied cognitions, we establish deep-seated beliefs about our internal reality. In a state of health, not only can we faithfully track our internal reality, but we can also reliably update cognitions about our body in tandem. That way, if our body becomes ill, then our mind detects the signals and forms new cognitions that our internal reality has changed for the worse. This process is critical because the updated cognitions prompt us to act. We might see a doctor or take a medicine or undergo surgery or talk to a therapist. But if the new cognitions never form, then our internal reality remains inaccessible to the mind's eye and we fail to address health threats. For patients like Diana, there is an urgent need to strengthen their interoceptive abilities. It turns out that virtual reality can help access internal reality.

Researchers from around the world are now using VR to break through the interoceptive blockade of anorexia nervosa. In a pioneering 2016 Dutch study led by Anouk Keizer from Utrecht University, a team of psychologists tested a VR body-swapping program in thirty women with anorexia.[10] Before using VR, they gave each participant a piece of string and asked them to loop it into a shape that represents the circumference of their hips and abdomen, but to do so without the benefit of checking against their own body dimensions. Then Keizer calculated the degree of misestimation between perceived dimensions and actual body dimensions. Next, the patients donned a VR headset and saw a first-person view of a normally proportioned female body. Using Ehrsson's body-swapping rules discussed in Chapter 1, Keizer convinced the patients they had fully embodied the healthy avatar through a combination of synchronized visual and tactile stimuli. Finally, after the illusion of living in a healthy body, the participants removed the VR headset and again estimated their body dimensions with the string.

The results were striking. Compared to a control group of women without anorexia nervosa, the patients with anorexia overestimated their body size prior to using VR. In some cases they were off by nearly double. This result was expected since previous research had also shown that people with anorexia misperceive their body dimensions. But after inhabiting a normally shaped VR body as if it were their own, the patients significantly reduced their body misperceptions and were more likely to portion off the right amount of string to represent their circumference. It's as though VR recalibrated their mind to acknowledge the true dimensions of their body. The authors concluded that "it is possible to decrease anorexia nervosa patients' overestimation of body size," and further emphasized that their study offered "important insights in the flexibility of body size experience in anorexia nervosa: It is not static and we can change it."[11]

Giuseppe Riva performed a follow-up study in a group of twenty-three patients in Milan, this time monitoring their outcomes for twelve months after the VR treatment. He also found that VR altered how patients perceive their body dimensions. But more important, Riva showed persistent cognitive and behavioral benefits a full year after the VR intervention. "We discovered that with just one session we were able to modify the experience of the body in these patients," he concluded.[12]

The Italian and Dutch research teams gained attention for their impressive results, but they are not alone. In 2018, a group of French researchers published a meta-analysis of studies using VR for eating disorders. After scouring the biomedical literature, the team identified twenty-six studies, including eight randomized controlled trials, evaluating the therapeutic benefits of VR. Although some of the studies were better designed than others, and despite some inconsistencies in the findings, the authors concluded that VR "is an acceptable and promising therapeutic tool for patients with eating disorders."[13]

To be clear, anorexia nervosa is a complicated disease that VR alone is unlikely to cure. Effective treatment requires a combination of psychotherapy, medical therapy, and dietary therapy sustained over months to years. There is no easy fix. But more and more, the evidence shows that VR is an effective adjunct to traditional therapy because of its unique ability to retrain the mind-body connection and enhance healthy body attention.

Under supervision from Riva's team, Diana received multidisciplinary care for her anorexia. It took thirty-seven sessions of intense intervention, but over time, she gained weight, improved her spirits, and learned how to reconnect her mind and body. On repeat testing, Diana was far more adept at detecting her heartbeat than she was at the start of therapy. Her interoceptive accuracy rose from 8 percent at baseline to 55 percent after treatment, a dramatic improvement that approached normal levels. And her interoceptive awareness? It fell from a score of ninety-four points at baseline to only seventy-one after treatment. This was not a regress. Rather, Diana's lower confidence reflected a healthy awareness that her mind and body had not been well coordinated; now that she acknowledged the deficit and learned to restore the connection, she was more cautious about her newfound awareness. According to Riva, these results "indicated that the extreme gap between Diana's perception and awareness of bodily sensations was partially and functionally restored at the follow-up assessment when Diana was not only able to correctly perceive her inner bodily sensations, but she was also able to better evaluate the correctness of those perceptions."[14] Diana's story proves something critical: interoceptive abilities are not static; they can be modified and trained.

VR helped Logan sense when his body was at ease, and it aided Diana in eating a more healthy and substantial diet. But what of the opposite end of the eating disorder spectrum? Can VR also help manage obesity by nudging the mind to consume fewer calories?

Obesity is a complex disorder with biological, psychological, and social determinants. Although there is no single explanation or optimal treatment for obesity, most people can lose weight when calorie intake is lowered to meet their basic metabolic needs. If we only ate when our body called for nutrition, then we'd support our physiologic requirements and avoid weight gain. But our desire to eat often has little to do with the physical demands of our body. We eat because it's social. Or we eat because we're bored or tired. Some people eat when they are depressed or anxious or need a distraction. In all of these cases, the drive to eat is dictated by more than nutritional needs; it is also dictated by psychological needs.

Giuseppe Riva believes the psychology of overeating relates to the mind and body falling out of sync. He theorizes that anorexia and obesity are both problems of diminished interoception, but with opposite consequences.[15] If anorexia results from the mind dismissing the physical burden of starvation, then obesity results, at least in part, from the mind neglecting the consequences of caloric overload.

Riva is using VR to reconnect mind and body with the goal of promoting healthier eating for people with obesity. In a 2016 case report, his team employed the same body-swapping technique used for patients with anorexia, but instead they applied it to a thirty-seven-year-old woman with obesity so severe that she needed a machine to help her breathe.[16] She had failed previous efforts at weight loss and was too unhealthy for gastric bypass surgery, an operation reserved for morbid obesity. Yet, despite the severe consequences of her illness, she continued to binge eat. Riva's team was called in to see if VR could help.

Just like with the Dutch anorexia study, Riva first asked the patient to estimate her body dimensions using a string. But in contrast to patients with anorexia who overestimate their body size, Riva's patient *under*estimated her size by half, indicating a profound distortion in body perception. He then used the VR body-swapping illusion to simulate a first-person perspective of a thin avatar. After inhabiting the weight-reduced body, the patient repeated her self-assessment and reported dimensions more in line with her actual size. She returned to her multidisciplinary care program, which had previously been unsuccessful, and subsequently experienced less anxiety about her condition and achieved clinically significant weight loss.

Encouraged by the success of a single case report, Riva expanded his research in a larger study of 163 women with morbid obesity.[17] He randomized participants to receive either standard behavioral treatments or VR-enhanced cognitive behavioral therapy. The VR program included fifteen weekly sessions designed to address the psychological

underpinnings of obesity. In one session, patients visited a virtual supermarket where they practiced shopping for healthy foods while skip-
ping past fattening treats. In another, they swapped into a thin avatar
and imagined feeling confident in a new body while lounging on a public
beach. Throughout the program, therapists worked with patients to recognize and manage emotional triggers for eating, practice temptation exposure in virtual environments, address perceptions about body size, and
internalize a feeling of control and competence around eating.

Riva found that patients lost weight during the immediate treatment period regardless of whether or not they received VR. But when
his research team returned a year later, they discovered major differences between the groups. Patients who received VR-enhanced therapy
were seven times more likely to have kept their weight off compared to
non-VR controls, most of whom returned to binge eating and regained
their weight. VR worked over the long term.

Halfway around the world at the University of Tokyo, another research team led by Professor Michitaka Hirose is also studying whether
VR can modify appetite. His team of engineers built "diet goggles" that
trick the brain into thinking the stomach is full by making food look
larger than it really is. In one experiment, Hirose instructed research subjects to eat an Oreo cookie while wearing a specialized VR headset with
forward-viewing cameras.[18] The cameras magnified the Oreo to appear
1.5 times its actual size relative to the user's hand, and then projected the
supercookie into the headset. When he asked participants to eat as many
Oreos as possible, they consumed 10 percent fewer cookies while wearing
the diet goggles compared to normal conditions without the headset. Of
course, the cookies didn't change at all; only the *perception* of the cookies changed. When Hirose ran the program in reverse and shrunk the
cookies down to two-thirds size, he found that people ate 15 percent *more*
cookies.

The Japanese team went a step further by rigging the diet goggles
with a bottle that deploys scents. Then they switched out the Oreo cookie
for a flavorless, low-calorie cracker, but continued to project a chocolate
cookie into the headset. As research subjects chewed the cracker, the

headset emitted a chocolate aroma to lend a sense of flavor. Eighty percent of people believed they were eating a calorically dense treat when, in fact, they were only consuming a plain cracker.[19] The scientists repeated the experiment with other stimuli, including a strawberry scent paired with a pink cookie, and a vanilla scent with a white cookie. No matter the combination, most people were fooled into thinking they were eating a tasty treat.

When a journalist asked Hirose to reflect on the implications of his work, he summed it up in one line: "Reality," he said, "is in your mind."[20]

Hirose's research reminds us that VR is a tool that modifies perception, and that perception becomes reality. When used to recalibrate unhealthy perceptions, VR can augment traditional therapy for many of our most pressing health threats.

Throughout Part I, we learned that when VR is used in the right way, for the right patient, and at the right time, it has potential to alleviate suffering. For conditions like anxiety and depression, VR can promote cognitive flow and help counteract the ruminating mind. For conditions like irritable bowel syndrome, fibromyalgia, or burn injuries, VR can dampen inner pain signals. For schizophrenia and dementia, VR can strengthen self-identity by enabling more organized thinking and by restoring a fractured sense of self. And for low interoceptive conditions, like anorexia and obesity, VR can enhance healthy body attention and help to restore mind-body connections. In all cases, VR can alter perception of the world in a way that, if done right, can improve lives.

But that's easier said than done. It's one thing to study the science of immersive therapeutics, but it's quite another to implement academic research on the front lines of healthcare delivery. There are barriers to using VR in everyday practice: VR doesn't always work; sometimes it causes side effects; headsets need to be sanitized; clinicians need training on how to select and implement the right virtual treatments; and administering VR costs time and money. In short, this isn't easy.

In Part I, we discussed the science of immersive therapeutics. In Part II, we explore how the science is reshaping the practice of medicine.

Virtual Medicine

I hope VR headsets will become kind of like toasters. Every home will have one, and even though you might not use it every day, it will be a practical form of media consumption. When that happens, a wider population of people will become familiar with VR and will come to expect it as part of their clinical care.

—Albert "Skip" Rizzo, PhD, director, University of Southern California, Institute for Creative Technologies

CHAPTER SIX

The Virtualist

"OH MY GOD, THERE'S MY GRANDMA!" EXCLAIMS HARMON CLARKE as he peers into his living room while lying in a hospital bed surrounded by an NBC News television crew.

"Good morning, Harmon, this is Nanna. I miss you."

Harmon is managing a severe case of Crohn's disease, an illness that has ravaged his body, mind, and spirit through intestinal inflammation and devastating infections. Harmon is only thirty-four years old, but he's already endured over thirty operations to remove large segments of diseased bowel, leaving him undernourished, often in pain, and dependent on a growing list of medications. Today he is trying something different to manage his disease—Harmon is traveling home to be with his grandmother and then visiting his favorite park to practice yoga, both of which he will do from his hospital bed.

At this moment, Harmon is wearing a VR device fitted snugly around his head. Twelve miles away, his grandmother sits in front of a baseball-sized 360-degree camera that's recording her house and beaming the images back to Harmon's hospital room where they are reconstructed into a perfect three-dimensional replica of her living room.

"Tell us what you're seeing," asks the news reporter.

"It's amazing. I feel like I'm sitting in my living room! Oh my gosh!" says Harmon, who normally lives with his grandmother when not confined to a sickbed.

Harmon knows he is sitting in a hospital room. His body feels the contours of his hospital bed and his ears hear the reporter asking questions from somewhere beyond, but his mind is elsewhere.

Next, he travels to the Kenneth Hahn State Recreation Area, a bucolic park in the center of urban Los Angeles. When he's not hospitalized, Harmon visits this park to practice yoga and mindful meditation. The 360-degree camera is now sitting beside a stream and recording the placid sounds of water cascading over smooth stones and the warbling of birds in nearby trees. Harmon takes notice.

"The breeze is blowing through, I'm sitting at the top of Kenneth Hahn park. And there's downtown, there's the Hollywood Sign . . . and there's my house!" he says, pointing at a pulse oximeter at the foot of his bed. "It's like I can smell the sounds. I can hear the sounds."

Notice his language. "I can *smell* the sounds." The experience is so intense that he exhibits a temporary form of synesthesia, where the senses are gloriously jumbled into a multisensory hodgepodge. This is not unheard of. Sounds in VR have a smell to Harmon, and why shouldn't they?

It is clear that Harmon is no longer in his hospital room. He now contorts his body into a lotus position, crossing his legs and holding his hands into the air, palms up. He is transfixed. The room is silent as everyone watches intently.

Having treated nearly three thousand patients with VR at Cedars-Sinai Medical Center, my research team has learned a lot about whether, when, and how to use immersive therapeutics for patients like Harmon Clarke.

Part I: Our Bodies, Our Selves showed that the science and research have matured. But knowing about the science doesn't necessarily mean that we're ready to use VR in everyday clinical practice. Sometimes, when I think back on my journey in immersive therapeutics, I wonder why I even thought to pursue this field in the first place. As the editor of a medical journal and a lifelong academic, I have read about countless biomedical innovations that didn't cause me to change my research focus. And as a Western-trained medical doctor, I had little formal training in mind-body medicine when I began learning about VR. Furthermore, as a nondigital native, I have even less knowledge about computer programming and gaming. It might not seem like an obvious decision to distribute video game goggles to acutely ill patients in the hospital.

But upon reflection, it turns out that using VR *was* an obvious decision for me; it was the inevitable consequence of technical, social, medical, and even political trends seventy years in the making. My research team happened to be in the right place, at the right time, and benefited from decades of buildup that made it acceptable to bring VR headsets into the hospital. In this chapter, I explain how it has taken a generation to set the stage for VR's ascendancy in healthcare. Acknowledging the historical context of immersive therapeutics provides a deeper understanding about why I believe that medical VR is here to stay and why I haven't quit thinking about it since that day in 2014 when I jumped off the virtual building. Technology constantly changes and advances, but the foundation of therapeutic VR is stable and robust.

I will start by considering my own institution, which is among the largest hospitals in the United States. Our hospital delivers outstanding care, but make no mistake about it, Cedars-Sinai, much less any hospital, is not a place of rest. Our patients can suffer grievously. They can suffer physically, emotionally, and socially.

Consider Harmon's daily routine. Each day begins with an early morning wakeup call, often at 5:00 a.m., where he is greeted with a needle stick to draw blood. His undernourished body resists the gesture. The technician struggles to find full, plump veins. This requires multiple sticks, each more painful than the last. Finally, he gets a moment of rest as the vials are whisked to the lab for analysis. But not for long. Just as Harmon drifts back to sleep he is awakened again, this time by a nurse to check vital signs and administer a pain pill. Dazed from lack of sleep and disoriented by brain fog, he lies on his back, stares at the fire alarm on the ceiling, and waits in suspended animation for the next interruption to arrive. Like clockwork, the doctors begin their morning rounds, marching in and out, poking and prodding, asking the usual questions ("How's your pain, Harmon? Does this hurt, Harmon? . . ."). Next, he's hauled off to radiology for a CT scan. Then he's escorted to the gastroenterology unit where he's sedated and a long tube with a camera is inserted and removed from his stomach. Finally, he is returned to his room, exhausted and distressed, where a tray of cold chicken broth and blue plastic-wrapped Jell-O awaits. Unsure of the time or even the day, Harmon stares out the window and watches cars crawl in traffic, birds circle in the distance, and palm trees gently bend in the wind. The world outside goes on without him as he lies in bed, stomach cramping, nausea rising, staving off sickness. Sleep. Finally. And then a new day begins with a fresh needle stick. The cycle continues.

I have been a doctor for over twenty years. It never gets easier seeing patients like Harmon suffer. Like many of my colleagues, as I progress in my career it becomes clearer to me that effective doctoring not only requires knowledge of anatomy and physiology but also demands attention to the emotional and social consequences of illness. We have to acknowledge the impact of disease on the whole person. We need to recognize that patients like Harmon not only suffer physically but may also experience emotional distress, social stigma, anxiety, depression, or a sense of isolation.

What do you value about your own health? What gives you a sense of well-being? As you contemplate these questions, you may find yourself considering physical, mental, and social aspects of health. Maybe you want to live as long as possible, but only if you can maintain meaningful relationships and physical independence. Maybe you are willing to live with a certain amount of pain or distress, so long as you can watch your children or grandchildren grow up. Or perhaps you would accept more physical pain if you could reduce emotional pain.

The United Nations grappled with these same questions when it formed in 1945. One of the first priorities of UN diplomats was to create a global health organization that could support all aspects of well-being. The result was the World Health Organization, or WHO, which formed to provide better healthcare for the world's citizens. In its 1948 charter constitution, WHO defined health as a "state of complete physical, mental, and social well-being, and not merely the absence of disease or infirmity."[1] With this landmark statement, WHO declared that human health has three components: *physical*, *mental*, and *social*. At a time in human history when empathy had reached rock bottom and tumult had dominated the world for over a decade, this tripartite model of health was remarkably forward-thinking and humanistic. It set the stage for a broader concept of health that acknowledges the interconnection between physical and emotional well-being.

Today, over seventy-five years later, the WHO definition of health remains unchanged. WHO has shaped public health policy and medical practice ever since its mid-century origins. For someone like Harmon Clarke, it means that doctors should do more than treat the inflammation in his colon or dull the throbbing pain in his belly. It also means they should treat the social anxieties associated with his condition, like not knowing if his ostomy bag might break and spill its contents while he's visiting friends. It requires they try to lift his spirits when things seem desperate. It requires they listen to Harmon, learn about what matters to him, and create a care plan that addresses his unique illness experience. It means they should think about him as a whole person rather than a patient with abnormal biology.

But in the second half of the twentieth century the practice of medicine began to deviate from the WHO vision of health. Remarkable discoveries in biology, genetics, and pharmacology enabled massive scientific advances that ushered in a new biomedical model that emphasized physical mechanisms of disease rather than emotional and social aspects of illness. According to this model, diseases had physical explanations and causes, and it was thought that most human illness could be explained by understanding the behavior of molecules, cells, tissues, organs, and body systems. Fixing the body would fix the patient. Psychology was considered a secondary discipline of unclear relevance to biomedical discoveries.

The biomedical model worked well for germ theory, for example, where eradicating bacteria could cure an infection like pneumonia. It was great for explaining how to fix abnormal body functions, like unblocking a clogged artery to stop a heart attack or healing an ulcer to treat stomach pain. It was an ideal model for explaining cause and effect, where problem A leads to disease B, and removing A cures B. It was a neat and tidy way of thinking about human health.

But it could not explain everything. Discoveries in basic science could not easily explain complicated interactions among one's health, genetics, environment, and illness experience. It struggled to predict why two patients with the same disease might experience vastly different symptoms, or why quality of life does not always correspond with lab test results.

In 1977, George Engel, a professor of psychiatry and medicine at the University of Rochester, proposed a new model of medicine that could address the insufficiencies of the biomedical model. He called it the biopsychosocial model.[2] In his treatise in the journal *Science*, Engel argued that medicine was in a state of crisis because the biomedical model was woefully shortsighted. He observed a prevailing belief that since disease was defined in terms of physical properties, doctors needn't worry about psychology because it lies outside the practice of medicine. Engel described a Cartesian mind-set among doctors that the body and mind were considered separate and apart, and that managing disease meant managing the body alone. This dualistic doctrine, he argued, was a shameful limitation of medicine and an abdication of physicians' responsibility to treat the whole patient.

Engel outlined an approach that still allowed for mechanistic interpretation of disease but also accommodated emotional aspects of illness. He proposed that medical doctors must gain expertise in social and psychological science, and he argued that addressing these components of well-being is perfectly compatible with the biomedical model.

Although initially met with some skepticism, Engel's vision took root. Doctors discovered that addressing all three components of health improved patient satisfaction and clinical outcomes. Moreover, doctors could provide holistic care without having to abandon their classical scientific training. Engel's powerful insight enabled a broader understanding that medicine is not about the false dichotomy of mind versus body, as Descartes proposed in the seventeenth century, but about integrating mind *and* body. This set the stage for the theory of embodied cognition, which we covered in Chapter 1. This theory later opened doors for VR to become a viable therapeutic intervention.

As the fields of psychiatry and neuroscience grew in the years after Engel's essay, it became evident that the brain is yoked to the rest of the body and governs critical functions well beyond its cranial boundaries. Noxious signals arising from the body, such as pain from cancer or an inflamed organ, could be controlled by modifying how the brain receives and processes those signals, as we discussed in Part I.

These discoveries ushered in a "beyond the pill" era in Western medicine that legitimized nondrug treatments. In the 1980s and 1990s, serious researchers began studying ancient practices like mindful meditation, yoga, and cognitive behavioral therapy. Studies demonstrated that these treatments are highly effective for a wide range of conditions, and in some cases more effective than traditional drug therapy.

Doctors also began to realize the importance of documenting how patients feel. Hospitals and clinics started to administer patient surveys and document the results in the medical chart. Patient perception moved to the forefront of medical decision-making. For example, you've probably seen this assessment tool in your doctor's office (I took this photo in my own clinic).

It was rare to find these emoticons in a hospital or clinic before 2001, when it became a national standard in the United States to document pain as a vital sign (in the next chapter we explore the unexpected

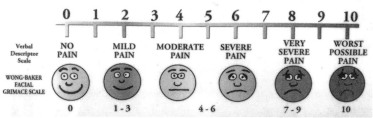

PAIN AND FUNCTION ASSESSMENT TOOL

This tool is intended to help patient care providers assess pain according to individual patient needs. Explain and use 0-10 Scale for patient self-assessment. Use the faces or behavioral observations to interpret expressed pain when patient cannot communicate his/her pain intensity.

0 1 2 3 4 5 6 7 8 9 10

| Verbal Descriptor Scale | NO PAIN | MILD PAIN | MODERATE PAIN | SEVERE PAIN | VERY SEVERE PAIN | WORST POSSIBLE PAIN |

downside of this practice). Then, in 2004, the National Institutes of Health created a sweeping program to measure patient symptoms across the human illness experience.[3] Now there are hundreds of questionnaires to track everything from fatigue to depression to joint pain. The 2010 Affordable Care Act legislated that healthcare providers measure patient experience in order to qualify for federal reimbursements. Doctors, clinics, and hospitals are now learning how to use these surveys to make better decisions.

As a result of these political and scientific initiatives, patients are now positioned at the center of clinical decision-making. It has become obvious why documenting the patient perspective is vital for clinical practice, just as Engel explained decades ago in his prescient commentary. In the forty years since his essay was published, medicine has transitioned from a "doctor knows best" mentality based in biomedical thinking to a model of shared decision-making that relies on the combined expertise of both patients and doctors to embrace all three WHO dimensions of health.

All this history brings us back to Harmon Clarke. His virtual escape from the pain of Crohn's disease was the result of a super-convergence of trends. First, if it weren't for the postwar enlightenment of WHO and George Engel's essay in *Science*, I might not have ever thought to introduce VR into Clarke's hospital room. I take it for granted to consider all three dimensions of health, but that's only because I was trained at a time when Engel's model was widely accepted and promulgated.

Second, if it weren't for modern advances in psychiatry and neuroscience, I might not have considered VR to be an acceptable therapy for hospitalized patients. I take it for granted that immersing patients in virtual environments can lift spirits and reduce pain, but that's only because thousands of my predecessors demonstrated the therapeutic benefits of other "beyond the pill" interventions across diverse fields of medicine.

And third, if it weren't for broad acceptance that emoticons matter in medicine, I might not have studied whether VR is truly impacting patient outcomes. I take it for granted to survey patient perspectives alongside checking lab tests and ordering X-rays, but that's only because social scientists developed patient health surveys, because measuring pain scores is now part of everyday clinical practice, and because legislators tied federal reimbursement to the results of patient questionnaires.

VR came at just the right time, and Harmon's lotus pose is the culmination of a seventy-year journey that brings us to today.

As compelling as Harmon's story may be, he is only one patient. Some of my more skeptical colleagues—mostly those trained in the biomedical model of medicine—still raise an eyebrow when they hear about VR. They have lots of questions: How do we know that VR improves health beyond individual anecdotes? How do we know that VR has an active ingredient and is not just an elaborate placebo akin to a digital sugar pill? And if VR does work in carefully controlled trials, as we saw throughout Part I, how do we know the results will carry over into the dynamic and messy environment of clinical practice? And then there's the issue of whether these treatments are cleared by regulatory agencies, like the Food and Drug Administration (FDA). I'll come back to that issue in Chapter 9.

Frankly, I had similar questions. I had experienced the presence of standing atop the building and could attest to the visceral nature of immersion. But I could not yet determine whether VR would make any difference in everyday patient care. I needed to run some of my own experiments. I needed to confirm this wasn't a case of irrational exuberance that a headset designed for virtual games could make a meaningful impact on real disease, in real patients, in a real hospital.

Our research team started by testing VR in hospitalized patients like Harmon. We knew there had to be a better way of lifting spirits than airing TV reruns of *The Price Is Right* or serving trays of neon Jell-O. We also knew that pain medications, like narcotics, might temporarily dull aches and dissipate anxiety, but that their benefits sometimes come at a steep cost of confusion, fatigue, and nausea, if not worse.

In our first clinical study we selected four VR experiences.[4] The first one, called *Paint Studio*, allowed patients to "paint" a virtual picture using head gestures to control the paintbrush. The second was *TheBluVR*, an underwater ocean adventure where patients could swim with blue whales, dolphins, and manta rays. In the third module, patients traveled to a Cirque du Soleil performance where they shared the stage with a cast performing graceful acrobatics. Finally, we offered *Tours of Iceland*, an aerial journey where patients flew in a helicopter over fjords, waterfalls, and geysers.

So we had chosen our hardware, picked out our software, and were ready to start testing.

Right off the bat, the science didn't translate neatly into reality. Many patients just refused to participate. That seemed odd to me. I wondered if there was something amiss about our recruitment procedures, or perhaps the consent language did not answer patients' questions. I decided to join our research coordinators to learn more.

The very first patient I approached was a forty-five-year-old woman who, a month before, had developed a "cold" she couldn't shake. It turned out she didn't have a cold at all; she had metastatic lung cancer without ever having smoked a day in her life. She had a young child and a supportive family at her bedside. I approached her with a set of goggles, explained how the VR might help with pain management, and described how the experience could offer a temporary escape from the hospital. She looked at me, silently and unblinkingly, as if I had dropped into her room from another planet. She politely turned down the VR, but I could see in her eyes that my request was out of place. I don't know if she would have reacted the same way if I had offered her a brilliant new pill, but it was clear she was not interested. I reflected on the fact that we were about the same age, yet I was upright and free while she was confined to the hospital. She died days later.

I tell this story because we cannot lose track of the very human element of healthcare when talking about a technology like VR. What may sound like a fantastical voyage to the well may seem like an unwelcome intrusion to someone who is in distress with an advanced illness. It is important not to overpromise and under-deliver on what technology can achieve in medicine. We'll come back to this issue in Chapter 8. In all my reading about VR in preparing to use it with my own patients, I had never come across a formal study about people refusing to try it. Nor had

I found case studies about the nuance of discussing VR with very sick patients who were concerned about simply surviving.

Two out of every three patients straight up refused VR in our first study. They never even made it into the headset. Many patients expressed skepticism, fear, or concern regarding psychological consequences or infection risk.[5]

One man was convinced we were conducting some kind of mind experiment. I remember him well. He was an older gentleman with a square jaw and cropped hair, sort of a military type. I offered him the VR goggles and he looked at me like I was crazy. "No chance," he said.

"Sure, no problem. Would you mind telling us why?"

"I didn't come here to be a subject in your psychology experiments. What's that thing do, anyway? Does it mind read? Can it tell you what I'm thinking? I can tell *you* what I'm thinking: Forget it. You can give it to someone else."

Understood.

Another patient couldn't be bothered to use the equipment. "I'm so weak and tired, the last thing I want to do is mess around with this stuff."

Others could not use VR because of medical or technical barriers. For example, some people experiencing nausea could not be safely placed in VR for fear of triggering cybersickness—a disquieting form of motion sickness triggered by feeling out of sync in the virtual world. Normally, when you move your head around it instantaneously alters your field of view. But if there is a delay between head movement and visual tracking, the brain gets thrown off and it creates unpleasant vertigo. Cybersickness is less common now that VR graphics are sharper and processing speeds are faster, but even the best VR systems can still cause this reaction. Since cybersickness can happen in people without illness, we thought it unwise to use VR in patients with nausea, dizziness, or vomiting; this decision meant that many patients were ineligible for the study. We will discuss cybersickness more in Chapter 8.

There were a handful of other shortcomings that became obvious only after working closely with patients. People with facial or head injuries could not safely place the headset over their wounds. Patients immobilized with neck fractures could not achieve presence because they were unable to move their head—all they could do was stare straight ahead or gently roll their body. For these patients, using VR was often more frustrating than therapeutic. Many patients in the intensive care unit had breathing and feeding tubes in their mouth and nose; navigating a headset around these vital devices proved difficult.

So our initial foray into therapeutic VR identified some barriers. We wrote them up and published the findings in a peer-reviewed journal so others could learn along with us.[6] I emphasize these limitations because they are real and must be addressed through more research and development. But I wouldn't be writing this book if the story ended here.

Among the first twenty-eight patients who tried VR at Cedars-Sinai, twenty-four had a positive experience, two were neutral, and two didn't like it.[7] That was an impressive debut considering the stress these patients were experiencing in the hospital. If a drug company invented a medicine that made 86 percent of acutely ill patients happy, then they would have a multibillion-dollar blockbuster drug.

One patient in particular stood out in the early phases of VR testing. Maria was a sixty-four-year-old woman with advanced liver disease. When the liver shuts down, it leads to painful fluid buildup in the abdomen, swollen legs, abdominal pain, confusion, and gastrointestinal bleeding. Maria had all of these complications and was hospitalized to manage her worsening disease. One day, I was walking through a medical ward holding a VR kit when a colleague saw me and asked if I might use it for Maria. He explained that the usual medicines weren't working and she was getting worse. The doctors could not easily control her pain and were unable to use opioids because the medicine would complicate her confusion. They were running out of options.

So Maria tried the VR. We selected *Tours of Iceland* for her initial experience. Off she went in the helicopter. As I watched her response, I noticed two distinct moments that seemed to indicate VR was working its magic. I've since seen this pattern repeat itself innumerable times. The first moment, which I call the moment of conscious immersion, typically comes within twenty seconds of use. This is the aha moment when patients become consciously aware they are within a broader, more expansive environment than initially recognized. When patients first don VR goggles and view the images, they often stare straight ahead, not yet recognizing the immersive nature of the experience. Some patients will discover this on their own, whereas others require prompting from the staff to move their head and explore the scene. But the moment they begin to move, there's a recognition that VR is different from anything they had experienced before. They almost always smile, laugh, or say something like "That's amazing!" It's at that very moment when patients recognize that VR is special and different. It is uplifting to witness the moment of conscious immersion; it is a brief respite of joy punctuating an often distressful situation.

The second moment, which I call the moment of physiologic immersion, typically arrives four to six minutes after initiating VR. Once patients are conscious of being in an immersive environment, the next step is for their autonomic nervous system—the part of the nervous system that operates without conscious control—to settle into the experience. Whereas the moment of conscious immersion registers in the higher cognitive centers of the brain, the moment of physiologic immersion is more of a brainstem phenomenon where the body automatically adjusts in rhythm with the experience. This is most evident when we use relaxing environments, such as a nature tour or a mindful meditation experience. We can actually see the *moment* the patient takes her first, deep, purposeful breath. The chest abruptly rises, then slowly falls, and the body posture changes markedly. The shoulders often fall back, the torso sinks deeper into the bed, and tension is released, all without conscious awareness. This involuntary physiologic cascade does not always occur, but when it does, as it did with Maria, we know VR is having a positive impact. We can see it without question. It's a beautiful thing.

After removing the headset, I asked Maria how she felt.

"Relaxed. Very relaxed," she said with a placid smile that belied the underlying disease plaguing her body. "I wasn't thinking about the pain. I was just thinking about being there and having a good time."

It's moments like this when I know VR matters. I've managed thousands of patients using countless treatments. But short of performing emergency maneuvers to restart someone's heart, I cannot think of many other treatments in my doctor toolkit that provide so much benefit in so little time as VR.

But how big is the benefit? And does it work better than a placebo? Or did people only like VR because of the way we presented the technology? Maybe patients felt obligated to like it to avoid offense. Or maybe VR was just a digital sugar pill. Remember, my more skeptical colleagues wonder if VR is voodoo science. As a dyed-in-the-wool academic, I also worried about whether there was sufficient evidence to promote VR for patient care. I had read the controlled trials, and so I knew VR outperformed all manner of control interventions across a range of conditions, but I still needed to see for myself. We have a saying in medicine: "See one, do one, teach one." I needed to see VR outperform a control intervention myself. If it could do that, then I'd be ready to do more VR, and teach more VR.

In our second study, we sought to answer these questions by testing VR in a new sample of hospitalized patients.[8] We separated them into two groups. The first group watched a 2-D video of relaxing nature scenes, including mountain lakes and running streams from Patagonian vistas along with an audio track of Native American shamanic music. We measured pain levels at baseline, ran the video, and then measured pain again to see if it changed.

The second group watched a VR experience called *Bear Blast* that was created to treat pain in patients who are bedbound or have limited mobility. This immersive game takes place in a bizarre fantasy world where users shoot balls at moving objects by maneuvering their head toward the targets. The scenes feature tribal masks floating in the sky and red gophers perched on ancient stone walls smiling manically and waving. It's just weird enough to grab your attention, and that's the whole point. In fact, it's super weird and super distracting. It kind of resembles the unbridled visions that people describe while tripping on psychedelics.

The results of the study were striking. Sixty-five percent of patients in the VR group reported a clinically meaningful drop in their pain after spending fifteen minutes knocking over gophers and blasting bug-eyed sky-masks. In contrast, only 40 percent of those in the control group had the same response after watching the 2-D relaxation video. That's a profound difference. By way of comparison, powerful opioids like morphine beat placebo by around 10 to 20 percent.[9] Our results implied that treating patients with a VR gopher-blaster might be better than using opioids, although we did not compare those treatments head-to-head. Importantly, we did not document serious side effects among patients in the VR group (more on adverse effects of VR in Chapter 8).

Buoyed by our success in the first two studies, we decided to conduct a larger and longer study.[10] This time around, patients in the VR group could use the headset whenever they wanted to slip it on—not just as a onetime treatment. They used VR three times per day, for ten minutes per session, and as needed for any bouts of severe pain. The patients then decided for themselves whether, how frequently, and for how long to use the VR. We offered a library of experiences, including a guided relaxation while lying on a beach, a visual poem depicting landscapes from the American desert, a ride on the Wright brothers' Kitty Hawk airplane, and an underwater swimming experience with dolphins, among many others. Patients in the control group viewed a health and wellness TV channel available in all rooms throughout our hospital. The TV programming included yoga and meditations, discussions about health and wellness topics, and poetry readings. This was a reasonable control condition because there is ample evidence that offering relaxation programming can reduce pain and emotional distress.

Because we were concerned that patients might prefer VR due to its novelty or as a consequence of unconscious preferences among the research staff, we designed the study to minimize response bias. Patients in both groups were informed that the study was testing the effect of "two types of audiovisual experiences" on the perception of pain. In order for the research personnel to exhibit equipoise when describing the competing interventions, we prepared a script that used neutral language regarding both interventions. In both arms of the study, we minimized investigator interactions with the study participants and relied on non-study nursing staff to collect pain scores. Patients used their assigned audiovisual experience on their own terms without a formal protocol. The study was designed to be a pragmatic assessment of VR compared to an active control condition already found in the treatment environment.

Once again, the results favored VR. Patients in the VR group experienced a nearly fourfold reduction in pain compared to those in the control group. We also discovered that patients with the most severe pain—that is, those with pain scores of at least 7 out of 10—had the most profound response to VR. It didn't matter what kind of pain the patient had—whether from cancer, gastrointestinal problems, orthopedic issues, or neurological pain—all types of pain got better with VR; it was indiscriminately helpful.

Overall, our experience in the hospital has shown that around 80 percent of patients have at least some kind of positive response to VR. There is now compelling evidence that hospitals should consider offering VR alongside opioids, sleeping pills, and antianxiety medicines. I believe it is time to expand the therapeutic options to include VR. It is also time to introduce a new type of clinician who is an expert in applying therapeutic immersive technology—the virtualist.

It's been two years since Harmon Clarke virtually left the hospital to visit his grandmother. Now he's standing on a stage before a sold-out audience gathered from around the world to hear his story. Harmon is a keynote speaker at Virtual Medicine, our annual course at Cedars-Sinai dedicated to training the new generation of virtualists.[*] He's holding up a VR headset and addressing the packed auditorium.[11]

"My name is Harmon Clarke," he begins, "and I'm here today because this device saved my life."

---

[*] To learn more about virtual medicine, visit www.virtualmedicine.health.

For an audience of technophiles, this opening statement commands attention. The auditorium is in rapt silence as Harmon begins his story. He explains that while growing up, he was a normal kid who played five high school sports, flirted with girls, and was a happy-go-lucky soul. Then he got sick. Things got worse. He went in and out of the hospital. Harmon recalls one especially frightful night:

"I had temperatures, fevers, chills, sweats, and hallucinations. I remember being in the hospital room and having two nurses hold me down as I screamed at night. I thought I was going to die. I remember being depressed and totally depleted. I thought, why is God punishing me?"

Harmon became desperate. He needed a way out, and fast. He wanted his old life back. The physical, mental, and social burden of his illness had become overwhelming. All three components of his health were suffering.

"My friends would come to the hospital every single day," he recalls. "As a kid, you naturally know how to escape. They'd come and play video games, cards, dominoes . . . whatever we had to do to get my head out of the hospital. I couldn't stay in that hospital. I couldn't stay in this place where death was surrounding me, or else I would give up."

That's how Harmon was feeling when our team first arrived with a VR headset. To Harmon, VR initially seemed out of place for such a severe disease. But then he discovered how VR could help him escape in a way he didn't expect. Harmon continues:

My pain got worse and worse. I was bleeding. I couldn't eat food. I was quarantined because my immune system was so low. The fear was overwhelming. I had no way to cope or deal with it other than the pain medicine, which would later lead to addiction. That's when the VR team came into my life. I remember them coming in with this big clunky device and these huge headphones, and them telling me this could potentially help with my pain and anxiety. And I remember thinking to myself, "You better get that out of my face, you have no idea what kind of pain I'm in right now. I need my pain meds." But

I had nowhere to go, so I figured I should just try it out. I had seen the commercials with people waving their hands. I'm like, this is good marketing, but like . . . really? Is this really how it works? So I put the headset on, and I remember being transported directly to Iceland. I was in a helicopter looking over waterfalls. I could feel the sun radiating on my skin. I could hear the birds chirping. And for those few moments, I wasn't in the hospital. This was the first moment I realized I could escape with something other than the pain medicines. I was taken away from my bed. I began working on breathing exercises. It helped me learn to meditate. Every night, it put me to sleep. Over the next few months I used VR like breakfast, lunch, and dinner. It was my go-to tool. I took my goggles with me everywhere I went. The VR showed me three very important things: that I could escape, that I could manage my pain using something other than opioids, and that I could use tools to help cope with my condition.

There are thousands of published studies on the therapeutic benefits of VR. There are hundreds of randomized controlled trials. There are even *studies of studies* summarizing the benefits of VR. I included over three hundred of these studies in *VRx*. The science is real. But there is no substitute for just hearing from patients. Harmon's story matters because it proves that the science of VR can translate from the pages of medical journals into the complex, messy, three-dimensional world of clinical reality. VR is not a panacea for grievous suffering, but if it can help people like Harmon through their darkest days, even if just a little bit, then we should make it available to more patients like him.

Yet chances are high that your doctor has never offered a VR treatment to you or to anyone else you know. There's a good chance your doctor has not even heard of immersive therapeutics. That is understandable, because it reflects the reality that the field is still evolving. The science may go back decades, but it is only recently that affordable, high-quality VR equipment has become available for clinicians to use with patients like Harmon. Moreover, any time a new treatment option emerges, be it medicine or machine, doctors tread carefully until they gain enough experience to feel comfortable with its use.

So we are at a crossroads. On the one hand, there is ample scientific and clinical evidence that immersive therapeutics work for people like Harmon. On the other hand, there are still very few clinicians who are trained to use VR in practice.

One day, Harmon and I got to talking about why more patients are not receiving VR treatment. We discussed the need for a clinical team solely dedicated to immersive therapeutics. That way, we could ensure that people who need it could benefit from VR without waiting for more doctors to obtain enough training and experience to feel comfortable using the technology. We also discussed how VR is not just a singular treatment, like a new pill, but rather is an extensible tool that cuts across healthcare. In this book, we note that VR is a treatment that applies to psychiatry, orthopedics, gerontology, gastroenterology, rheumatology, neurology, dentistry, dermatology, pain management, obstetrics, and pediatrics. We'll also look at its applications in even more specialties, such as cardiology, rehabilitation medicine, ophthalmology, and neurosurgery. Because VR is more than a single treatment, it is not straightforward for doctors to just start using VR like they might with a new medicine. VR is far more than a new treatment. It's a new treatment paradigm.

Talking with Harmon helped me realize that in order to scale immersive therapeutics across healthcare we need to train a new class of providers who are VR authorities. These virtualists not only will be experts on the latest hardware and software but also will understand whether, when, and how best to integrate VR within Engel's biopsychosocial framework of health. They will be highly skilled and multidisciplinary clinicians who work in partnership with specialists to augment traditional therapies across a wide range of conditions. Virtualists will balance breadth and depth: they will be deeply knowledgeable about the treatment paradigm of VR, including its risks and benefits, but will apply that paradigm broadly across disciplines. In Chapter 8, we explore the risks of VR. Then, in Chapter 9, we discuss how virtualists can optimize the benefits of VR by following the "three rights": prescribing the *right* immersive therapeutic, to the *right* patient, at the *right* time. In Part III: Brave New World, I project how virtualists will impact the practice of medicine for years to come.

But first, let's see how VR can translate outside the hospital to manage one of the greatest health threats of our time. It is an epidemic that pulled in Harmon, too.

"There was still another hurdle that I had to overcome," Harmon tells the virtualists-in-training as he concludes his speech. "When I tried to stop the pain meds they started in the hospital it was just horrible. The chills, the sweats, the shaking. So I had to seek professional help. I checked into a drug rehab center to get help for my condition. And I'm happy to say that I haven't had to take pain meds since, and I've kept off of them because of the mental tools I gained from using VR."

Can VR help others with opioid use disorder? Or is Harmon's story unique? Unbeknownst to Harmon, at nearly the same time he discovered VR while in the depths of pain and despair, another man facing the battle of his life also turned to VR to help fight his way out.

CHAPTER SEVEN

Fighting the Opioid Epidemic

Robert Jester looks like he came straight out of a Norman Rockwell painting. A beloved schoolteacher from Greenport, New York, Jester has a contagious smile and a kindly face. True to his community roots, he is both a volunteer fireman and the local chimney sweep. One day working atop a chimney in the summer of 2016, Jester fell to the ground and broke nineteen bones in his body. He was airlifted to Stony Brook University Hospital in Long Island where doctors placed three rods and sixteen bolts in his fractured spine. When he woke up, he found himself paralyzed below the waist.

Jester's accident would change his life forever. For the next year, he endured multiple surgeries, engaged in year-round physical therapy, and used medicines to dull the pain in his damaged body. "I didn't think a human could experience this much pain," he told me in an interview while sitting in his wheelchair. "That's the only way I can describe it."

The pain invaded his sleep. It affected his mood. It kept him down. All the while, he continued taking oxycodone—an opioid medication in the same family as morphine and heroin—to stave off the suffering. He began to realize the painkiller was causing physical and mental dependency. On top of that, he knew opioids sometimes cause digestion problems, trigger psychological distress, and disrupt normal sleep patterns. In some cases, opioids have the paradoxical effect of worsening pain over time—a phenomenon called hyperalgesia, where escalating doses yield diminishing amounts of pain control. Despite past promises from drug companies that opioids are minimally addictive substances, those claims have proven to be demonstrably and tragically false.[1] Jester knew better, too.

"The science teacher in me was always concerned about the pain medicine because I was taking so much of it," he said. "I forced myself just constantly to fight every day to take less, and less, and less medication."

Jester started experimenting with drug-free techniques to reduce the pain. He had heard about the research using VR for pain control and thought it worth a try. He began a daily regimen of immersive therapeutics that included meditating on a beach and traveling to Machu Picchu. "If I was having real serious pains and felt like I wanted to take another Oxy, I'd strap on my headset. It turned my attention away from the pain."

VR allowed Jester to wean off the opioids. He took what he learned in virtual reality and used it to combat pain in real reality. "In VR, I learned that my mind has some control over the pain. I figured out how to hone that control so I could use it even when I wasn't in VR. That way, I'd still have pain relief for an hour or two after I used the headset." After several months of VR treatment, Jester cut the opioids for good. "I don't even have Oxy in the house anymore," he told me. "I used up my last pill and never renewed the prescription."

Jester's story of suffering and opioid use is all too common. There are fifty million people in the United States with chronic pain, a human toll that surpasses the prevalence of diabetes, heart disease, stroke, and cancer combined.[2] But unlike Jester, many people cannot pull themselves out of opioid dependency. There is an urgent need to learn from his story because America is in the midst of an opioid epidemic that demands timely and effective solutions.

If a full 747 jumbo jet were to crash every three days, year-round, then the catastrophic toll would equal the nearly fifty thousand people who die annually from opioid overdoses in America.[3] You might imagine this could never happen to you or a loved one. But here's something to ponder: Let's say you've never used opioids before and now your doctor prescribes a short-term treatment of Vicodin or OxyContin for a dental procedure or a sprained ankle. It's a routine treatment that happens every day of the week, all around the country. There's nothing to worry about, right? You fill the prescription in the pharmacy, take it home, and swallow the first pill. You continue taking the medicine for the rest of the day, exactly as instructed, and you find that it indeed reduces your throbbing pain.

What is the chance that you will still be taking these pills a year later? By then, your discomfort should be long gone, so you wouldn't expect to still be swallowing painkillers. The Centers for Disease Control and Prevention (CDC) examined this question and calculated the answer: There's a 6 percent chance of dependency a year after a single day of use.[4] But what if you take the opioids for ten days? By then, your risk of dependency rises to 14 percent. And it only goes up from there. By the time you get to a month of use, your chance of long-term dependency closes in on 30 percent. And once you're dependent, the risk of all-cause mortality nearly doubles compared to before starting the drugs.[5]

Where did this epidemic come from? Humans have known since the Neolithic age that the yellow-brown latex inside the opium poppy has medicinal properties. Every ancient society, from the Greeks to the Sumerians, widely employed opium for religious and therapeutic purposes. The ancient Sanskrit word for poppy literally means "magical." Once scientists learned how to extract and concentrate the active ingredient of poppy seeds, which is morphine, doctors could offer metered doses for patients in both the operating theater and the theater of war. It also became clear that opium is highly lethal; it has been used for euthanasia and poisonings. The history of opioids is a complex tale of science, warfare, economics, religion, politics, social hierarchies, and world culture.[6]

Flash-forward to 1961 when the United Nations ratified the Single Convention on Narcotic Drugs treaty. This treaty, which is still supported today by over 180 partner states, regulated the production and distribution of opium and a growing list of synthetic look-alike compounds such as hydrocodone, oxycodone, and fentanyl.[7] It was the first worldwide proclamation that opioids pose serious risks to human health. In the United States, the Controlled Substance Act of 1970 fulfilled America's obligations to the UN treaty by specifying how regulatory agencies would monitor the prescribing of opioids. Expectations were set. Laws were passed. And then, for a while, prescribing went largely according to plan. There was a healthy appreciation among doctors that opioids, albeit highly effective when used appropriately, must be used with caution for fear of causing dependency, morbidity, and death.

Things changed on January 10, 1980, when a modest 101-word letter to the editor, titled "Addiction rare in patients treated with narcotics," was published by two Boston University authors in the vaunted *New England Journal of Medicine*.[8] The brief report, which underwent no formal peer review and lacked scientific details, stated that "although there were 11,882 patients who received at least one narcotic preparation" in the Boston University Medical Campus records, "there were only four cases of reasonably well documented addiction." And with that one result, the authors summarily concluded that "despite widespread use of narcotic drugs in hospitals, the development of addiction is rare."

This single, unsubstantiated report became a rallying cry for doctors and drug companies that it was now safe to prescribe opioids. Comforted by the finding that only a tiny fraction of hospitalized opioid users would ever become addicted—at least according to a five-sentence letter in the back pages of a medical journal—prescriptions skyrocketed. Somehow, one short and dubious report was enough to overthrow millennia of history bearing witness to the destructive power of opium and its derivatives. The letter was so influential that it prompted a follow-up study in 2017 by scientists at the University of Toronto, also published in the *New England Journal of Medicine*, that reviewed the impact of the original letter on the arc of the opioid epidemic.[9] The study found that the letter had been cited in 608 scientific publications during the thirty-seven years since its release, and that most of the citations indicated the letter offered "proof" that addiction is rare among opioid users. The authors of the 2017 study concluded that "this citation pattern contributed to the North American opioid crisis by helping to shape a narrative that allayed prescribers' concerns about the risk of addiction associated with long-term opioid therapy."

If the Boston University report was the kindling for the opioid epidemic, then the conflagrating spark was the release of OxyContin by Purdue Pharmaceuticals in 1996. Also called Oxy for short, OxyContin is a long-acting form of oxycodone originally thought to be safer than short-acting "quick hit" opioids like morphine; it's also the medicine Robert Jester used before turning to VR. For ten years after Oxy's release, Purdue made strong and consistent marketing claims that its product was safe and minimally addictive. The company treated doctors and their families to luxurious retreats, bought them lots of trinkets, and in return, seemed to expect a quid pro quo rise in prescriptions. They even created a promotional video called *I Got My Life Back* that profiled inspirational stories of Oxy curing severe pain. Purdue sent fifteen thousand copies of the video to doctors around the country to use as waiting room freebies. The number of opioid prescriptions rose by eight million between 1995 and 1996 alone. In the mid-1990s, the total opioid prescription volume was roughly 100 million, and by 2012 it reached a peak of nearly 300 million. To be sure, Purdue's scandalous marketing was partly responsible for this increase. In 2007, in the midst of the opioid wave, three senior executives at Purdue pleaded guilty to federal charges that they misled the public about the risks of OxyContin. But it took years after this legal victory before anyone could begin to slow the epidemic of prescribing opioids that Purdue and others had been cultivating for over a decade. By 2019, Purdue agreed to pay up to $12 billion to settle legal claims and then filed for bankruptcy.

It wasn't just doctors and drug companies that fueled the opioid epidemic. The federal government and regulatory bodies also fanned the flames with a set of ill-conceived policies. In 2001, the Joint Commission on Accreditation of Healthcare Organizations designated pain as the "fifth vital sign" to be routinely measured alongside heart rate, respiratory rate, blood pressure, and temperature. This was a big deal, because the Joint Commission is the definitive accrediting body for more than 21,000 US healthcare organizations; when the Joint Commission says something, people in healthcare listen. Because accreditation is required for hospitals to receive federal reimbursements, passing the Joint Commission inspection is a top priority. Opioids were prescribed liberally to stay in compliance with the Joint Commission standards. What purportedly began as a humanitarian effort to focus needed attention on pain management evolved into an inpatient prescribing culture driven by a perverse incentive to perform well under the watchful eye of the Joint Commission. I say "purportedly" because the Joint Commission justified their 2001 standard in a book doctors could purchase for continuing medical education seminars. The book claimed "there is no evidence that addiction is a significant issue" with opioids, and confidently assured readers that contrarian views were "exaggerated."[10] And guess who sponsored the book? Purdue Pharmaceuticals. The Joint Commission subsequently removed their discredited standard in 2009, two years after the Purdue executives were found guilty in federal court.

When I graduated from medical school in 1998 I knew very little about opioid prescribing. It was barely covered in our curriculum beyond basic pharmacology. Outside of prescribing opioids for advanced cancer, my professors did not emphasize their use. I heard more about physical therapy, psychotherapy, and mind-body treatments than I did about narcotics. This period in the late 1990s coincided with the rise of George Engel's biopsychosocial model. Yet, by the time I graduated from medical residency in 2001, I was prescribing opioids left and right in the hospital. We all were. By 2004, when I finished advanced training in gastroenterology, I witnessed a collateral epidemic of opioid-induced constipation, also called OIC, that triggered a cottage industry of medications to treat the side effects of opioids—meds to treat meds. More than a decade later, I no longer prescribe opioids,* but I still do prescribe OIC drugs to manage the digestive consequences of opioids.

The opioid epidemic is far from over. The fallout comes in unexpected ways. A few years ago I was called in by doctors to use VR for a patient with uncontrolled pain who was on morphine. When my team arrived with the headset, the patient had already died of unexpected respiratory failure, a possible consequence of the opioid.

But the tides are changing. In the past several years, the federal government enacted a set of initiatives to stem the epidemic. The CDC published new opioid guidelines in 2016 that pushed doctors to be more responsible prescribers. The FDA placed black box warnings on oxycodone and fentanyl that strongly caution about the risk for abuse, addiction, overdose, and death. Also in 2016, Congress passed the bipartisan 21st Century Cures Act that allocated $1 billion in funding to expand treatment and prevention programs for opioid addiction. In 2018, the National Institutes of Health (NIH) announced $1 billion in earmarked funding to support new science and treatments for managing chronic pain. The initiative, called Helping to End Addiction Long-term (HEAL), included funding for pain-fighting technologies that offer patients and doctors drug-free alternatives for battling pain.[11] Our team was fortunate to receive funding through this program to support our VR research. Then, in March 2020, I was invited by the FDA to discuss the science of VR analgesia. For VR researchers, this blast of funding and regulatory interest is like wind in the sails for charting new scientific progress. The stage is now set for a scientific renaissance in immersive therapeutics for pain.

In Chapter 3 we learned that VR dampens pain signals via three effects: distracting the brain through inattentional blindness;

---

* Although I do not prescribe opioids in my practice, I do believe many people meaningfully benefit from responsible use of these medicines. I also recognize that people who take opioids can be unfairly stigmatized, adding insult to injury. There is still a role for using these medicines. When opioids are indicated, I refer patients to pain specialists who are skilled in safely managing these prescriptions.

fast-forwarding pain through time acceleration; and blocking pain through gate control. But the examples we discussed mainly focused on managing acute pain for short-term experiences like childbirth, episiotomy repair, needle sticks, dental procedures, colonoscopy, or burn dressing changes. We also need to know whether VR can help with *chronic pain*—not just acute pain—from relapsing conditions like fibromyalgia, chronic regional pain syndrome, or recurrent neck and back pain. What is the evidence that other people like Robert Jester with long-standing pain can also achieve some relief from virtual worlds? To answer this question, we need to first distinguish acute pain from chronic pain.

Acute pain is an appropriate and time-limited response to tissue damage. If you get stuck with a pin or put your hand near a hot stove top, then your pain nerves fire, the signals pass up the spinal cord, and your brain registers the "ouch." This continues until the damage heals and the nerves stop firing. Then the pain goes away and you return to normal.

But chronic pain is different. In some cases, like with Robert Jester, the tissue injury takes time to heal and the pain signals continue to bombard the spinal cord and brain. Over time, this nonstop stimulation leads to pain sensitization, where the nervous system exaggerates pain signals beyond what is appropriate for the amount of physical injury.[12] It's as though the body accepts a new mission to warn the brain of imminent danger despite there being little or no threat. In the spinal cord the pain signals are amplified and shot up to the brain with greater frequency, intensity, and duration than would otherwise normally occur. The unabated pain signals inundate the brain, causing anxiety, depression, and mental distress. The brain loses control of its defenses and no longer blocks the pain effectively. The result can be a vicious cycle of worsening pain even after the original injury is long gone.

These changes can become semipermanent if they are not stopped. Our central nervous system is "plastic": its structure and function can change over time, for better or for worse. As the spinal cord and brain continue to withstand a salvo of pain signals, the nerves begin to rewire themselves. The pain gates in the spinal cord swing open and stay open.

The nerves keep firing, even without a persistent injury. The result is unflagging pain, anxiety, depression, sleeplessness, exhaustion, irritability, and worst of all, diminished ability to do anything about it. People become helpless and hopeless. The psychic pain can be more overwhelming than the physical pain. Anyone who has felt this kind of pain knows the depths of suffering a human can sustain.

Ronald Melzack, co-originator of the gate control theory, offered this stark assessment of chronic pain in a scholarly overview written with Joel Katz, a psychologist at York University in Toronto:

> Most backaches, headaches, muscle pains, nerve pains, pelvic pains, and facial pains serve no discernible purpose, are resistant to treatment, and are a catastrophe for the people who are afflicted. . . . Pain may be the warning signal that saves the lives of some people, but it destroys the lives of countless others. Chronic pains, clearly, are not a warning to prevent physical injury or disease. They *are* the disease— the result of neural mechanisms gone awry.[13]

So acute pain and chronic pain are very different. Acute pain is a normal response to a noxious stimulus. Chronic pain is a disease unto itself. VR might work for acute pain, as we saw in Chapter 3, but can it make a dent in chronic pain?

Diane Gromala has been thinking about this question for the better part of three decades. A professor of computer science and design at Simon Fraser University in British Columbia, Gromala began a quest in 1991 to study how VR could manage chronic pain. Her background is like few others in the field of immersive therapeutics. In addition to holding a PhD in computer science, earning a master's degree in fine arts from Yale, and working at Apple in the early 1980s where she honed her skills in software design, Gromala has also suffered from chronic pain since early childhood.

Gromala has tried it all when it comes to managing her pain, but that doesn't stop people from offering her unsolicited advice. "So, invariably when I meet someone and I tell them I have chronic pain," she said in a

TED Talk, "I hear them ask *'Have you tried . . . ?'*" And then she flashed a slide with over fifty pain remedies, including acupuncture, transcendental meditation, hot stone massage, colon cleansing, magnetic bracelets, ashtanga yoga, primal scream therapy, and, of course, opioids. "Yes," she said, *"I have! All of it!"*[14]

Gromala combined her expertise in art, design, and computer science to create immersive experiences for people with chronic pain, starting with herself. Her insight was that VR could teach patients how to tame their inner turmoil. She did this by equipping patients with biosensors to measure subtle body cues that are normally imperceptible. For example, she used tiny sweat sensors to monitor moisture in the skin, which she calls the "mood ring of the body." Even minor changes in sweat levels can reflect the earliest signs of stress. Gromala also measured breathing rate, blood pressure, and heart rate to capture other physical responses to stress. She fed the data back into a VR headset, where an iridescent blue jellyfish swam around in lockstep with the streaming data. As the patient breathed in and out, the jellyfish synchronously pulsed to propel itself forward. As stress levels began to drop in the patient, the jellyfish progressively dissolved to nothingness and the visual field went black. This had the effect of promoting biofeedback-enabled introspection. In essence, patients learned how to reduce the traffic passing up their interoceptive highway, just like the examples noted in Chapters 3 and 5.[15]

Gromala's team used this technique to create a so-called meditation chamber where people could learn to control their pain in a virtual environment.[16] She demonstrated that VR taught patients to slow their heart rate and reduce the moisture in their skin. The technique worked especially well for those who had never before meditated, suggesting it was an effective way to introduce newcomers to the practice of mindfulness. "People had a sense of mystery solved about their body," Gromala explains.

By coupling VR to biosensors, Gromala offered patients a new level of mastery over their emotions, ultimately leading to new cognitions about the nature of pain and the ability to control it from within. "VR is a mirror for interoceptive senses," she says. "It tells us something about how our inner states and sensations work. It helps us understand the ways in which our wet inner world—these enormous universes within—can be tapped for curative purposes. And that's an idea that I think is worth spreading."

Gromala tested her meditation chamber with over four hundred research subjects, including herself. When I met with Gromala to discuss her research, she was quick to explain that VR biofeedback does more than merely distract from pain. It has a more durable effect of allowing patients to manage their pain long after removing the headsets, likely through blocking pain at its source. "They learn to exert some form of control or agency in their experience of unrelenting pain," she explained.

The results from Gromala's work jibe with earlier evidence that perceived controllability of pain strongly affects the neural response to pain. In a 2004 study by a team of neuroscientists at the University of Wisconsin–Madison, Tim Salomons and colleagues exposed research subjects to painful heat stimulation and monitored their brain response using fMRI.[17] Half the time the subjects were told they could control the duration of pain using a joystick device, and half the time they could not manipulate the pain. As it turns out, the joystick didn't work; it only offered a *perception* of controllability. Nonetheless, when people thought they had control, their fMRI showed lower activity in key brain areas that govern interoceptive pain. In other words, Salomons showed that interoception could be modified just by *thinking* it could be modified. Gromala leveraged this finding by offering direct access to unconscious inner signals using biofeedback, and then she employed her sensor data to drive a metaphorical visual narrative. In doing so, she brought the unconscious inner world to life in a way that could be seen and consciously manipulated.

In a 2016 follow-up study, Gromala's team performed a randomized study with chronic pain patients using a VR game called *Cryoslide*.[18] Participants spent ten minutes sliding through icy caves and throwing snowballs at peculiar creatures, much like Hoffman and Patterson's work with burn patients that we discussed in Chapter 3. One of the creatures was called a "neuron tree," and it looked like a shrub with red eyes, sharp teeth, neuronal dendrite-like arms, and a mean streak. The metaphorical concept of *Cryoslide* is to destroy the source of chronic pain by busting up the dendritic creatures before they get out of control. The study showed a 37 percent reduction in pain intensity with VR—a value that was greater than achieved with non-VR distraction techniques in the control arm of the study, and also a larger response than is typically achieved with opioids.

Other researchers around the world are discovering similar benefits of VR for chronic pain. For example, Hilla Sarig Bahat and colleagues at the University of Haifa in Israel tested VR for patients with chronic neck pain to see if it could improve cervical range of motion.[19] As someone with a chronically stiff and painful neck ever since an early-life whiplash injury, this study caught my attention. The investigators recruited patients with neck pain and divided them into VR and non-VR groups. The VR group entered a virtual environment where flies buzzed around their heads incessantly (talk about a pain in the neck . . .). Patients in the VR game had to "spray" the flies by pointing a target that was affixed atop a virtual spray canister. The position of the canister was determined by head motion, so people with a limited range of motion had to extend themselves to shoot the flies as they circled farther and farther away. The study found that patients in VR achieved a significantly broader range of motion both in terms of rotation and flexion-extension movements of their neck. They also moved faster and smoother, based on sophisticated measurements that were obtained up to seven days later to confirm the response lasted beyond the immediate treatment. The authors concluded that the immersive quality of the VR motivated patients to achieve greater mobility with less pain compared to non-VR controls. An Israeli VR startup company called XRHealth created a commercial version of the game where, instead of tracking bugs, the user follows dragons that are flying around a castle. I gave it a try and achieved an improvement in my neck flexibility based on objective measurements using a range of motion scale embedded within the software.

Beyond neck pain, other researchers have shown benefits of using VR for fibromyalgia, chronic migraine headaches, phantom limb pain, spinal cord injuries, and complex regional pain syndrome. I include references for all of these conditions in the back of the book.[20] On balance, the research so far demonstrates that VR can help manage chronic pain and improve functional performance. However, the studies have been limited to short intervals with limited follow-up. Before we can make any real promises about the benefits of VR for treating chronic pain, we need more studies that monitor patients not only for hours or days, but for weeks, months, or even years. We need to know if VR can slow the transition from the symptom of acute pain to the disease of chronic pain. And we need to know if the academic science translates to the frontline battles of the opioid epidemic.

Ted Jones knew his community was in trouble when the local government erected a public "overdose memorial Christmas tree" to honor families who lost loved ones to a drug overdose. Jones tells me about the public tribute from his office inside the Pain Consultants of East Tennessee in Knoxville, where he personally treats over five hundred patients per year for chronic pain.

"It was like a body count memorial for our community," he explains. If the opioid epidemic has a geographic center, then it's not far from Knoxville, Tennessee. In 2017, the Knoxville memorial Christmas tree had 247 ornaments, one for each community member who died from an overdose in the previous year.[21]

"Then there are the near misses," he continues. "Last year alone, first responders in Knoxville administered emergency naloxone over twelve hundred times."

Naloxone is an injectable drug that reverses the effects of acute overdose by blocking opioids from binding with their target receptor. It can save lives, but only if it's administered fast enough. Pain doctors are distributing naloxone far and wide to arm their communities with this vital antidote. Cities like Knoxville track naloxone use as another barometer of the opioid epidemic.

"In Knoxville, we give out naloxone to the police, to the paramedics, and to family members of our patients on opioids. In some other communities even librarians are trained to use naloxone. There's a disproportionate number of opioid deaths in public library bathrooms, so librarians are now first responders," he explains.

Jones looks down at his clasped hands and shakes his head. "Then there are the babies. The children's hospital in Knoxville created a whole new wing just to deal with neonatal abstinence syndrome, or NAS, where babies are born already dependent on the opioids and need to be weaned off." The opioid epidemic literally rebirths itself every day in Knoxville, and in thousands of other cities and towns throughout America.

Jones and his colleagues have seen enough.

"We need solutions now. This is an emergency. We can't wait any longer. We need effective painkillers that are not addictive and can replace opioids."

As a pain specialist, Jones had been following the therapeutic VR literature for a while. He was aware of Hoffman and Patterson's research using VR to manage acute burn injuries, and Jones wondered if VR could also help his patients with chronic pain. He decided to perform a study and publish the results, however they might turn out.[22] Jones partnered with Firsthand Technology, a VR company in San Francisco whose founders worked on the original *SnowWorld* program, to test another of its therapeutic pain products called *COOL!* Similar to *SnowWorld*, *COOL!* guides users on a journey through an interactive and highly distracting fantasy landscape. Rather than snowmen and penguins, *COOL!* features otters amid caves, hills, and forests. And rather than throwing snowballs, users toss fish at the otters who move about in a playful way and change colors when struck. The developers are quick to emphasize that there is no violence involved (no otters were harmed in the making of *COOL!*).

Jones recruited thirty patients with severe, chronic, and unremitting pain from conditions ranging from spinal issues to shoulder problems, digestive disorders, and fibromyalgia, which is a common and burdensome disease that manifests with pain throughout the body. Unlike patients in the acute pain VR studies, these patients had lived with pain for an average of sixteen years, with one patient enduring forty-three years of pain.

They were fifty years old on average, so this was not a group of digital natives. Jones measured the patients' pain just before administering VR, then measured it again during the treatment, and finally repeated the pain assessment soon after finishing.

He recorded a 60 percent reduction in pain between the baseline measurement and first measurement while in VR, and a 33 percent reduction after the treatment was completed. One in three patients reported 100 percent relief during the VR session. In a follow-up study, Jones repeated VR sessions with *COOL!* on a weekly basis over the course of one month to test whether its benefits were sustainable.[23] Each week, patients came back for VR treatment and reported their pain scores. This time, he found a 53 percent average drop in pain from the VR. Moreover, the pain relief did not immediately wear off. Jones observed what he called an "anesthesia tail" that lasted an average of thirty hours after turning off the VR. He found this residual effect in 90 percent of his patients. One person said the benefit lasted for seventy-two hours.[24] Jones also found no evidence of habituation—that is, the benefits of VR remained stable week-in and week-out.

Other research supports Jones's findings. One study by Charles Rutter and colleagues at the University of Maryland evaluated the benefits of VR for experimental pain over eight consecutive weeks.[25] Each week, the research subjects returned to the lab where their hands were dunked in ice cold water—a painful stimulus—both with and without VR. The study again revealed that VR reduced experimental pain, but it also found that the benefit did not diminish with reexposure. Hoffman and Patterson found the exact same thing when repeatedly treating burn patients with VR.[26] It seems that the pain-fighting benefit of VR does not easily wear off. Opioids, in contrast, often yield less and less benefit and may require higher and higher doses to maintain the same effect over time.

I asked Jones to place all this research into a broader context.

"Well, it's like this," he explained. "Morphine cuts pain by twenty-five to thirty percent on average. We found that VR cuts chronic pain twice as much as morphine, does it with far fewer side effects, and doesn't exhibit the same habituation and tolerance that we see from drugs."

These are promising conclusions. Nonetheless, Jones did not study VR in a head-to-head trial against opioids, nor did he test whether VR reduces the amount of opioids needed to maintain adequate pain control. For VR to make a difference in the opioid epidemic, we need evidence that it is powerful enough to replace painkillers. Robert Jester and Harmon Clarke were both able to quit meds with the help of VR, but they are only two people.

Hoffman and Patterson conducted the first known experiment pitting VR directly against opioids.[27] In their forward-thinking study published in 2007, the same year Purdue executives were charged with stoking the flames of the opioid epidemic, the research duo was busy studying whether VR might one day replace, or at least reduce, the need for opioids. They recruited normal healthy subjects and placed them in an fMRI brain scanner. Then they touched their skin with a nondamaging hot probe and measured the response. The investigators repeated the experiment with VR alone, then again using an intravenous infusion of hydromorphone (Dilaudid), and yet again using a combination of both VR and hydromorphone at the same time. They found that VR achieved the same pain reduction as the powerful opioid infusion, and also discovered that both caused similar changes in the brain on fMRI scanning. Not only did VR calm the areas that process pain signals in the brain, but it also quieted the emotional centers that worry about those signals. With this striking result, Hoffman and Patterson demonstrated equivalence between VR and opioids. Then, when VR and Dilaudid were combined, the pairing was more powerful than either therapy alone. The authors concluded that VR might serve as a substitute for opioids in some patients, or possibly as an adjunctive therapy for those who have severe pain requiring opioids but who need to lower their doses. VR might also allow people who are starting a new course of opioids to begin on a lower dose with less risk of causing long-term addiction.

Just south of Washington State at The Oregon Clinic in Portland, a more recent study by Theresa McSherry and colleagues directly tested the opioid-abatement hypothesis.[28] These investigators performed a randomized trial using *SnowWorld* among hospitalized patients who required painful wound care procedures. This time, in addition to measuring pain scores, they quantified the amount of intravenous opioids required by patients in VR versus non-VR conditions. The study revealed a 39 percent reduction in fentanyl use when patients used VR. This was a meaningful short-term reduction in meds; these findings offer more evidence that VR can help to avoid the opioid.

In the wake of McSherry's research demonstrating opioid-level benefits of VR, coupled with other studies showing that VR can lessen the dose of powerful painkillers,[29] more and more clinics and hospitals have chosen to deploy immersive therapeutics in their own local opioid battles. At my medical center, we had already seen VR work for pain management in a hospital setting, but we didn't yet know if it also worked once people left the medical center. We decided to give it a try.

I am standing on sunbaked clay in the middle of a foreboding landscape. To my left is a gnarled and leafless tree. Above me is a violet sky filled with thunderclouds. A crow caws somewhere in the distance, punctuating the ghostly breath of wind blowing in my ears. Directly in front of me is a large, oblong crystal floating a few feet above a ceremonial stone altar. The crystal slowly bobs up and down but never touches the ground. It's as if the crystal is held in place by a tractor beam. The crystal is glowing red hot and radiating a sphere of dark energy. Now, a woman with a calming voice begins to offer me instructions.

"Using your breath, cool down the crystal so it can sustain life and energy again," she says. "Exhale slowly. Focus on your breathing."

I breathe in through my nose, noticing the cool and dry air as it passes through my nostrils. Then I slowly breathe out, focusing on the warm, slightly humid air that emerges. I watch as my breath releases into a stream of sparks directed at the crystal, where it strikes its glowing hot surface and vaporizes into steam. The crystal briefly dims and turns blue in response.

"Breathe out in a peaceful way," she instructs.

I continue breathing in and out, trying to cool off the levitating, red-hot crystal. The scene begins to change after a minute of focused effort.

The tree to my left has grown leaves. The sky brightens as the sun rises beyond a distant mountainscape. The sound of wind is replaced by a drumbeat.

"Exhale slowly. Focus on your exhales. Release your tension. Surrender to your breathing. The whole world is breathing with you now."

I look over to that tree again, and now the leaves are colored a brilliant shade of pink. The tree expands and contracts in rhythm with my breathing, like a huge arboreal lung exchanging air in sync with my body. The crystal has turned a lustrous shade of blue. The clouds have parted, leaving an azure sky mixed with a tangerine hue from the horizon. A mourning dove flies past my left ear. The scene is coming to life. It borders on psychedelic.

"Enjoy the relaxation you feel. Enjoy the soothing air leaving your body."

The drumbeats get heavier and a chorus of voices lends an ethereal tone. The sun is burning bright now. If I look closely, I can make out solar flares shooting off its surface. The crystal is also shimmering, like it's about to blow. Green sparks are pouring off its surface. And then, in a climactic fit, the crystal emits a bright field of light and a giant mandala fills the sky indicating some cosmic achievement.

"The crystal is holding energy again."

And then, fade to black.

I have experienced just one of more than fifty VR modules in *EaseVR*, a program designed for people struggling with chronic pain. In this segment, called "Cooling Crystals," pain is metaphorically stored in the smoldering stone and then dissipated into the environment with the help of mindful breathing. The microphone embedded in the VR headset tracks respirations and enables cognitive flow—that ecstatic state we explored in Chapter 2—through the help of meditative biofeedback. In other modules, patients can meditate on a beach, breathe vibrant colors into a black-and-white landscape, and learn diaphragmatic breathing skills in a forest.

Treating chronic pain is about more than dulling nerve endings. It's more complicated than that. Using a drug like morphine might lower pain temporarily, but it doesn't teach patients how to manage their pain or how to address unhelpful cognitions about pain. In contrast, *EaseVR* teaches skills that patients can take with them outside the headset to help them break the opioid habit or lower the chances of starting meds in the first place.

Josh Sackman is the cofounder of AppliedVR, the company that developed *EaseVR*. Sackman founded his company with the sole purpose of leveraging VR for health benefits like pain reduction. After five years of programming, testing, and studying the pain literature, Sackman and his team emerged with *EaseVR* as their first major product. One of their earlier programs, called *Bear Blast*, was the subject of my own clinical trials I discussed in Chapter 6. Now, Sackman and his team are in my lab showing us their latest software. One by one, our team members are transported from a conference room to virtual pain-fighting worlds.

"Pain usually goes hand in hand with anxiety and depression, so if we're going to treat chronic pain, we also need to treat comorbid mental health issues," Sackman explained. "When we designed *EaseVR*, we studied the principles of cognitive behavioral therapy, which we know helps with anxiety, depression, and pain, and applied these principles to VR."

You may recall from Chapter 4 that we discussed VR-enhanced cognitive behavioral therapy, or CBT, for managing schizophrenia. There is also evidence that CBT works for pain.[30] With CBT, therapists teach their clients to find ways of restoring meaning in life, even in the face of pain. They emphasize that physical pain is an inevitable part of life, but suffering is optional. Rather than dwelling on pain, CBT replaces unhelpful ruminations with new activities that bring value, meaning, and purpose. For example, people in pain often feel like their symptoms flare up just by thinking about them. They may be consumed by fear anticipating when the pain might occur next, or they may think constantly about what situations might bring it on. Other people in pain may want to eliminate suffering completely or return to an earlier state of better health, but that's not always possible. CBT attempts to change the mindset that pain must be extinguished, and instead offers strategies to avoid suffering.

In CBT, therapists might even ask their patients to trigger discomfort on purpose—by tightening their painful muscles or pressing on their aching back—and then observe whether the negative consequences really appear as expected. Studies show that when people attempt to activate the very symptoms they fear—pain or otherwise—they often gain improved symptom management and greater control over their illnesses. This highlights the distinction between pain and suffering. The pain might be unavoidable, but the suffering is the mess surrounding the pain—the worry, the obsession, the fear. When people allow themselves to confront their pain, they often find that it's not as bad as they expected, and they might regain control over the experience. Based on this research, a Silicon Valley startup called CognifiSense created a VR experience where patients can see their own body, identify the throbbing areas, and blast away the pain from the perspective of a disembodied first-person shooter. Another company out of Kentucky, called BehaVR, allows patients with pain to fire away at words flying around in space, with the goal to knock out negative sentiments and preserve the positive sentiments.

Sackman had CBT in mind when he designed *EaseVR*. Using the program is like having a personal therapist instructing you on how to redirect distressing thoughts, breathe with your diaphragm, and distinguish pain from suffering. But rather than receiving pain-directed CBT in an office or clinic, patients using Sackman's program experience CBT in a neon-infused dreamscape within the comfort of their home. And that part is key: if we are going to make headway with the opioid epidemic, we need to go beyond the hospital and go to where people live. Bringing VR home can help promote lasting change for a recalcitrant problem like chronic pain. We also need effective, home-based CBT programs that build skills through training and practice, because reprogramming the brain takes time.

We decided to test a virtual CBT intervention in our outpatient clinics at Cedars-Sinai. We developed a "digital pain reduction kit," which included a headset with *EaseVR* along with a library of other therapeutic experiences, including swimming with dolphins, strolling through the Redwood National Park, sitting beneath the aurora borealis, meditating on a beach, and playing the *Bear Blast* pain distraction game.

The kit also featured a device called a transcutaneous electrical nerve stimulator, or TENS, which is a small, battery-powered unit with electrodes that stick to the skin and deliver low-grade electrical impulses to nerve fibers. TENS causes a slight buzzing or tingling that feels comfortable, almost like a light massage. The science of TENS is based on the observation that people scratch a bothersome itch or rub their elbow after bumping it on a table. By stimulating the area around a trouble spot, we were trying to run a distraction along the nerves and close the pain gates in the spinal cord, thereby reducing bothersome signals from reaching the brain. Although the scientific literature on TENS is somewhat conflicted, it is an FDA-cleared technique that is safe and widely accepted.[31] So we supplemented VR with TENS in the hopes of achieving therapeutic synergy, meaning that using both together might be stronger than using either treatment alone.

Both techniques are thought to release natural opioids in the spinal cord. You read that right. *We are all equipped with an inner painkilling pharmacy.* You may know of endorphins, which are hormones secreted by the brain and spinal cord that activate opiate receptors, causing natural pain reduction. As a lifelong runner, I've experienced the "endorphin rush" countless times. For me, the effect typically occurs between forty and forty-five minutes into a run. That's when I feel a transition from tension to fluidity—from arduous work to pleasurable flow. I don't know what it is about that time window, but for me it's a near constant. It feels good.

Endorphins are among a class of natural substances that activate our opiate receptors and calm our nerves. Another natural opioid is called enkephalin, which closes the pain gates in the spinal cord. Enkephalin is like the morphine of the central nervous system. When it is released, enkephalin bathes the opiate receptors and inhibits transmission of pain signals in the spinal way station. If we can use non-opioid therapy to coax out our natural healing opioids like enkephalin, then we may have a way to reduce suffering, improve quality of life, and save costs without the need for more pills. At least that was our theory behind the digital pain reduction kit.

But does it work? That's the billion-dollar question. The research shows that VR works in the short term for both acute and chronic pain.

We have also seen evidence that VR can reduce opioid use after short bouts of therapy. But we need more data on the long-term benefits of CBT-based VR for chronic pain. Our trial with VR and TENS combination therapy is a multiyear study that will take time to complete. Other hospitals around the world are conducting similar research.

Our very first patient in the study offered hints as to what might happen. We enrolled a twenty-three-year-old man after he sustained a fracture to his forearm while riding on an e-scooter (as an aside, I've seen a lot of serious injuries from e-scooters). We approached him in the hospital after his surgery and provided him with the digital pain reduction kit and detailed instructions. We spent a good hour reviewing how to use the components of the kit. He seemed to get it and took the equipment home after being discharged. One week later our research assistant gave him a call. The conversation went something like this:

"How are you doing?"

"I'm doing okay. I'm still having pain but getting along."

"How's the virtual reality working for you?"

"The what?"

"The virtual reality? You know, the goggles that you wear to help distract your mind from the pain."

"I'm not sure what you're talking about."

"Do you remember we gave you a bunch of equipment to take home with you to help manage your pain? There's a set of goggles and a device called a TENS unit that sticks on your skin to help with pain."

"Oh . . . right. I saw that stuff in my room but didn't remember what it was for. Should I be using that for something?"

And so on.

As it turns out, when we met with this patient in the hospital, he had taken so many opioids that his brain fog clouded out the entire conversation about the VR. He was on meds, in distress, recovering from a serious injury and a surgery, and evidently was not in a state of mind to retain details about using a bunch of electronics. The research assistant reviewed it all with him on the phone. Then, a week later, we called him again.

"How are you doing?"

"Great! I love the VR! It's really helping me control the pain. I love how I can focus on my breathing when the pain flares up, or swim with dolphins under the water."

So, on the one hand, VR seemed to be working. But on the other hand, it only worked when it was actually being used. We learned from this experience that we cannot just drop a bunch of technology on patients and expect they will use it, even for digital natives. We also learned that human coaches really matter, because they augment the effectiveness of immersive technology. For that reason, we now employ a digital health coach who calls each patient once a week to check in, troubleshoot the technology, confirm adherence, and answer questions. The health coach learns something valuable from nearly every phone conversation, which allows us to fine-tune our approach to immersive therapeutics.

Time will tell whether our ongoing clinical trial reduces long-term pain and opioid use. In addition, more hard-fought science is required to determine whether hospitals and insurance companies should adopt VR for injured patients like Robert Jester. But one thing is for sure: If VR is going to work long term to help combat the opioid epidemic, a delicate balance between person and machine is required. It will obligate a unique brand of humanistic healthcare. It will mandate that we engage patients meaningfully in their own care and ensure they view immersive technology as a therapeutic extension of mind and body, not as a temporary, short-lived fix for pain. We will return to this topic in Chapter 10.

CHAPTER EIGHT

Primum Non Nocere

THERE IS A COMMON DICTUM IN MEDICINE, PRIMUM NON NOCERE, OR "first, do no harm." Every medical student learns this phrase early in training. It's often repeated in hospital wards and clinics as a reminder to be thoughtful when prescribing a treatment, performing a procedure, or undertaking a surgery. As a doctor, it's my job not to harm a patient. But inevitably, even the very best intentioned, most skilled, and most experienced doctors cause harm. In 1999, the Institute of Medicine published a groundbreaking report, titled "To Err Is Human," that concluded up to 98,000 people die each year from preventable medical errors.[1] That's more people than die from colon cancer, Alzheimer's disease, or the opioid epidemic. If we lose that many people to human errors, then one can only imagine how many near-death experiences occur or, for that matter, how many people sustain nonfatal side effects of care.

Risk-free medicine is a myth. Primum non nocere is at best aspirational. Drugs have side effects. Surgeries can sometimes make things worse. Talk therapy can summon dark and painful memories. In 2001, Dr. Kenneth Lecroy penned a widely read editorial in *American Family*

Physician debunking what he called "the outdated lie of primum non no-cere." In it, he wrote that physicians "need to allow our patients to understand why and how it is no longer possible to 'first, do no harm.' For every patient I have seen," he said, "I have had to rewrite the law. Every drug used, every prescription written, and every procedure has risk."[2]

When doctors utter that Latin aphorism, what they really mean is benefits should, on average, outweigh harms when making medical decisions. The art of medicine is about how to balance the evidence of risks and benefits, how to communicate that balance to patients and their families, and how to make shared decisions that optimize health while limiting harm. "It is only in *not* doing," Lecroy writes, "that we can give a 100 percent assurance that we will not harm."

VR is very safe compared to just about any other medical treatment. But even VR can and will do harm, sometimes, and to some patients. James Spiegel, a professor of philosophy at Taylor University who has written about the ethics of VR, points out that technological innovations like VR can be a mixed blessing. For all the benefits of VR that we've examined up until this point, there are also physical, psychological, and moral hazards posed by the technology. Spiegel views VR adoption as a "Faustian bargain, a trade-off where something good is gained while some other good is lost. And just as the positive aspects of VR are significantly great, so are the negative aspects."[3]

This chapter is about why VR can cause harm and how to mitigate its risks. We'll begin with an unlikely discussion about tiny crystals and fluid-filled tubes inside our head. From there, we'll learn how VR not only can trigger adverse effects on the body by messing with those crystals and tubes but also how it can produce existential effects on the mind.

Forty years after Descartes christened the era of mind-body dualism, another French scholar was busy recording scientific observations about the human body. A celebrated physician and member of the Royal Academy of Sciences, Guichard Joseph Duverney was best known in his time for public anatomical exhibitions in Paris, including dissecting an elephant before King Louis XIV. But it was not his work on great beasts, but rather on the minuscule anatomy of the inner ear that earned Duverney his scientific fame.[4] In 1683, Duverney trained his microscope on three semicircular tubes hidden inside a tiny lacuna deep within the skull. The tubes were curiously oriented at perfect right angles to one another, as though aligned in perpendicular X, Y, and Z planes. Duverney surmised that the planar orientation helped to maintain balance. If the tubes didn't work, then people might feel dizzy, nauseous, or off-kilter.

The exact function of the tubes remained shrouded in mystery for a century until Antonio Scarpa, an Italian anatomist, reexamined the inner ear with a higher power microscope previously unavailable to Duverney. As he peered through the lens, Scarpa spied a most unexpected discovery: tiny sacs of stones. When he traced the length of each semicircular tube, he noticed they were filled with fluid and terminated in a bulbous microchamber. Within the chamber were sheer-faced stones, like multifaceted crystals in an impossibly small treasure chest. This sighting only deepened the mystery. Scarpa remained unclear about how the tubes worked but proposed their mechanism must somehow relate to those minute bags of rocks.

As microscopes became even more powerful and scientific techniques more sophisticated, the perplexing tubes began to reveal their secrets. In 1892, the German anatomist Ernst Ewald made yet another breakthrough discovery: the fluid in the tubes sloshes back and forth in synchrony with head movement. He determined that hydrostatic forces keep track of head position in space. Now the anatomy made sense; the tubes are arranged at right angles in order to capture all possible motion within a three-dimensional coordinate system. Shake your head left and right and the fluid in the horizontal tube tracks the movement. Nod up and down and a second vertically oriented tube detects that displacement. Move your ear toward your shoulder and, sure enough, a third tube sloshes its contents in synchrony. Ewald had revealed an amazing bit of microengineering.

But what about those tiny crystals? It turns out the stones bob up and down in the sloshing fluid like buoys anchored in the ocean. When the weighted crystals jiggle about, they trigger specialized nerve endings to inform the brain about balance, position, and acceleration. This explains why you feel dizzy after spinning around in place. Once you stop, the fluid in your inner ear keeps moving, causing the tiny crystals to float up and down in the inertial waves. Your brain is convinced that you are still moving when, in fact, only the fluid is still moving—not you.

In the mid-twentieth century the burgeoning aerospace industry took interest in these discoveries about the inner ear. It's one thing to feel dizzy while on the ground, but quite another for it to happen while flying a plane or spacecraft; spatial disorientation can have life-or-death consequences in these high-stakes environments. But unexpectedly, it wasn't actual flight that caused issues with the inner ear tubes—it was *virtual* flight that made people sick. As computers became faster and graphics more realistic, pilots began training in simulators where they sat in a mock flight deck and watched a virtual scene through a windshield. Simulators were effective for rehearsing maneuvers, but they left some pilots feeling ill—sometimes very ill. In the original flight simulators created by Bell Aircraft Corporation for the US Navy, where pilots sat in a fixed chair and watched a moving scene, more than half the airmen felt nauseous, dizzy, or exhausted after a training session. It was not uncommon for pilots to unceremoniously vomit in the midst of virtual flight even though they were not literally moving anywhere. The problem was serious and common enough to earn a name—simulator sickness, or sim sickness for short.

Almost immediately after VR systems became available to the public outside of military or research applications, consumers began complaining of the same inner ear symptoms as navy pilots in the early flight simulators. People who rarely felt sick while playing 2-D video games became nauseous, dizzy, and fatigued after playing in immersive 3-D environments. This VR-related form of sickness earned its own unique moniker: cybersickness.

Motion sickness has historically been one of VR's greatest threats to adoption. Even if there are benefits from using VR, nobody wants to feel nauseous and dizzy. As the VR industry expanded, developers recognized that minimizing cybersickness was vital for sustained growth, not only because vertigo caused users to permanently discontinue use but also because financiers required that developers address the problem in order to justify further investments.[5]

Thankfully, VR companies worked to meet the challenge. Whereas VR cybersickness occurred in over 10 percent of users in the past, it has become less common thanks to dramatic improvements in hardware and software. More powerful computers enable faster visual frame rates, meaning more images per second. This is important because the slower the frame rate, the worse the feeling of sickness. Also, when the processing speed of the computer is slow there can be a delay between head movement and perceived movement of the VR image, a phenomenon called latency. Closing the sensory gap helps align the eyes with the inner ear. Other technical advances have reduced eye strain, minimized physical discomfort of wearing the headset, and reduced unnecessary visual motion. All of these efforts are making cybersickness a less prevalent and less serious problem. Mild symptoms are usually short-lived and improve with adaptation over repeated sessions. Severe cybersickness, on the other hand, can be very uncomfortable and may not subside until after a good night's sleep. Severe cybersickness now occurs in less than 5 percent of my patients using VR. But it still remains an issue. Although severe symptoms are rare, mild or moderate cybersickness is more common and can still reduce a patient's willingness to continue using VR.

In the meantime, as technical fixes continue to evolve, VR developers should also become more rigorous about testing for cybersickness prior to disseminating their programs. Natalia Dużmańska, a psychologist at Jagiellonian University in Kraków, Poland, authored comprehensive guidance for developers to consider when creating VR treatment programs.[6] Dużmańska encourages testing for cybersickness early and often using the Simulator Sickness Questionnaire, a validated checklist that measures physical side effects of VR. The questionnaire covers everything from nausea to visual problems to disorientation. If everyone used this screening tool, Dużmańska argues, then the medical VR community would have a common standard for judging the safety of new programs. We would expect the same for any drug therapy, so it makes sense to mandate the same level of rigorous monitoring for virtual therapy. In Chapter 9 we explore how often this really occurs and discuss how regulatory bodies like the FDA are starting to take note.

But it turns out that VR can do more harm than causing dizziness and nausea. As more and more people gained experience using VR, reports began to surface that it could also induce bizarre psychological symptoms. Testimonials emerged of VR triggering altered states of consciousness, not unlike Mel Slater's virtual out-of-body experience, where people described floating in a dreamlike state detached from themselves and others. Some recounted a disturbing sense of losing their identity, and still others felt like they had departed reality altogether.

Let me tell you a story of the first time I really encountered the dark side of VR.

Gloria had been experiencing abdominal pain for years by the time she reported to the emergency department for help. A twenty-eight-year-old stage and television actress, Gloria had become so ill that she could no longer remain on set long enough to complete her scenes. Her doctors tried all sorts of treatments, from antidepressants to stomach acid blockers to dietary changes. Nothing worked. Medical tests failed to identify a clear-cut cause of her pain.

The emergency department staff saw that she was in distress, so they admitted her to the hospital where, as is customary, Gloria underwent even more tests to diagnose her pain. Once again, everything was negative. The doctors called in my team for assistance. Gloria seemed like an ideal candidate for immersive mind-body therapy because her scans had not yet found a clear-cut source of pain, suggesting a possible stress-related problem. Maybe VR could help to reveal a cause.

Gloria was willing to try it out. We decided to use *Bear Blast*, the pain reduction game I described in Chapter 6. It seemed like a benign choice; what could be harmful about tossing balls at teddy bears in a fantasy world? In our clinical trials with *Bear Blast*, we recorded a 24 percent reduction in pain across a range of conditions, including the type of abdominal pain Gloria was experiencing.

For several minutes she politely wore the headset but didn't seem engaged. She appeared more like a passive observer than an active participant.

"You can see the whole world around you if you move your head. Feel free to explore."

"Yes, I understand," Gloria replied, continuing to stare straight ahead.

"Okay, great. Just let us know if you have any questions."

Another minute passed. She wasn't having a good time. She seemed detached from the experience and maybe even upset. But it was hard to tell since the mask obscured her face.

"Everything okay in there?" I asked.

No response. In the past, when people didn't respond to my questions while in VR, it usually meant they were lost in thought or too distracted to hear. But this time felt different because of her blunt affect and minimal engagement.

"Are you okay?" I repeated. Nothing.

And then she started to cry. Her body shook, her hands trembled, and in one fell swoop she tore off the headset and threw it across the bed, revealing a wide-eyed look of distress. She was hyperventilating and shaking.

"Make it stop!"

Bear Blast had triggered a full-blown panic attack.

It took us a few minutes to work Gloria through her distress. We didn't yet know what had happened, so we focused on reorienting her to reality and offering headspace to sort through the experience. In a situation like that, asking too many questions can worsen the panic. We instead focused on trying to help her breathe slowly and deeply, relaxing tense muscles, and thinking about positive memories and feelings. It took a bit of time, but Gloria was able to settle her mind and body long enough to reflect on what happened.

"I don't like violence," she said. "It brings back really bad memories."

This was surprising. Our VR library, and indeed most immersive therapeutics, deliberately avoid violent content. But as it turned out, the problem was that our notion of violence was too narrow.

"It made me sad to hurt the bears. I don't want to hurt anyone, even those bears. I knocked them over. I wanted to stop it but I couldn't. I had no control. I kept hurting them."

Our team had used *Bear Blast* many times before without anyone mentioning this concern. To most people, tossing balls at teddy bears is silly fun. But not to Gloria. She proceeded to describe a history of physical, emotional, and sexual abuse tracing back to childhood. We sat in silence as she recounted the horrors. She explained how even the slightest suggestion of violence, especially if she was the provocateur, evoked dark memories. *Bear Blast* made her feel like an aggressor. She knew exactly what those bears were feeling. She cried for them, then panicked upon realizing *she* was causing them pain.

To my surprise, Gloria said she wanted to try again, but she wondered if we had another, more calming experience. We were reluctant, but we reviewed our menu of options to see if any stood out. She stopped me when I mentioned Cirque du Soleil.

"That's it. I want that one."

And so we tried it. Gloria found herself on the stage of Cirque du Soleil among the performers. She watched and listened to the sights of acrobats dangling from ribbons and the sounds of the orchestra. Just like the first time, she sat quietly and passively, not showing signs of engagement. But then, after about a minute, she started to cry again. This time there were tears of joy. She was smiling ear to ear.

"It's so beautiful," she said. "I love it!" Gloria explained how the VR made her feel courageous. She said that, as an actress, her strength comes from standing on a stage. "I am powerful as a performer. I feel strong in here."

Within minutes, Gloria went from the depths of panic to the heights of ecstatic flow. We arrived at a possible cause of Gloria's abdominal pain—her years of abuse—but also triggered distress along the way.

To understand how throwing balls at teddy bears can trigger a panic attack, we need to think about how VR not only can trigger physical disequilibrium, as it does with cybersickness, but also how it can cause mental distress.

Rebecca Searles, a journalist who specializes in digital media innovations, wrote a 2016 article in *The Atlantic* titled "Virtual Reality Can Leave You with an Existential Hangover."[7] In it, she revealed emerging stories of VR's bewildering aftereffects. Searles recounted how Lee Vermeulen, a video game developer, was mid-conversation with a colleague after trying a VR demo when his mind went off the rails. "While standing and in the middle of a sentence," said Vermeulen, "I had an incredibly strange, weird moment of comparing real life to the VR. I understood that the demo was over, but it was [as] if a lower level part of my mind couldn't exactly be sure. It gave me a very weird existential dread." In another online post discovered by Searles, a VR user pleaded for help to diagnose his friend, who experienced a peculiar reaction to virtual immersion: "He started saying that he was feeling strange, a very odd feeling, not physical but psychological. . . . He said that it was something hard to describe: something like the concept of being in another world, another reality. . . . It was like anxiety but still related to the feeling of being in another distinct reality."[8] With her compendium of stories, Searles exposed a new and troubling side of VR. "It seems that VR is making people ill in a way no one predicted," she concluded.

In one notable blog post, titled "The Post Virtual Reality Sadness," Tobias van Schneider, a popular game designer, described a post-VR experience he called The Derealization that occurred after he recovered from the immediate vertigo of cybersickness:

> I start to feel better physically. Objects seem to be normal again, I don't feel dizzy or anything. . . . But what stays is a strange feeling of sadness & disappointment. . . . The sky seems less colorful and it just feels like I'm missing the "magic." . . . [In VR] I feel like god for a couple hours, with magical and powerful tools right at my finger tips. I can do anything I want! After leaving a world like this, the rest of the day in reality makes me kind of sad. I have no more super powers. I want to touch the sky, rotate the clouds, stretch them and paint on them. I feel deeply disturbed and often end up just sitting there, staring at a wall.[9]

There is precious little research examining the mechanisms of post virtual reality sadness, as van Schneider calls it, but what literature exists again implicates, at least in part, those tubes and crystals in the inner ear—what scientists call the vestibular system.

In 2015, Kathrine Jáuregui-Renaud, a Mexican neuroscientist, published a paper summarizing the evidence linking inner ear function and depersonalization/derealization symptoms, also called DP/DR for short.[10] *Depersonalization* means feeling disconnected from oneself, such as having an out-of-body experience. *Derealization* is the feeling of being disconnected from reality, as though living in an alternative time or place than is objectively true. DP/DR symptoms fall on a spectrum with prolonged daydreaming on one end and dissociative disorder on the other, a clinical condition where people are deeply absorbed into their imagination, leaving them feeling detached from themselves and their external world. Subclinical DP/DR symptoms are common, occurring in up to 25 percent of people sometime during their life. Such symptoms are so prevalent that psychologists believe some degree of DP/DR is normal and might have evolved as an escape from the occasional brutalities of reality. This would explain why DP/DR is commonly reported under extreme life-threatening circumstances.[11] But when DP/DR happens without warning, or when it can't be controlled, the result is distressing. It can cause downright panic.

In her scientific review linking DP/DR to the inner ear, Jáuregui-Renaud revealed that when there's a mismatch between senses, as occurs with VR cybersickness, it becomes difficult to interpret reality. The world feels off-kilter. It's like when you are sitting in a stationary train and feel a sense of movement because another train outside the window is pulling away. When sensory conflict occurs in someone already susceptible to DP/DR, the result can be alarming. For this reason, Jáuregui-Renaud recommends testing for DP/DR *before* putting someone through VR. This straightforward procedure, which involves administering a short questionnaire, can help determine whether to use VR, and if so, which software to employ. We will return to this idea of personalizing therapeutic VR in Chapter 9.

Jáuregui-Renaud's research indicates that the semicircular tubes and crystals do much more than track head position. The brain also uses their signals to process emotions, cognitions, and sense of self. According to Jáuregui-Renaud, the inner ear signals are a critical ingredient for selfhood; they convince the brain of its physical location and support the sense of embodiment. Without perfectly timed signals from the inner ear, the brain begins to question whether it owns the body to which it is connected. The result is a peculiar sense of Cartesian dualism, where the mind feels separated from the body. It's so distressing because it is so unnatural.

It is this insight—that the inner ear informs our embodied sense of self—that begins to explain how fooling the vestibular system not only can cause cybersickness but also might trigger psychological consequences like a panic attack. Beyond Jáuregui-Renaud's research, additional evidence supporting this finding traces back to 1998 when a group of Harvard psychologists published a paper titled "Dizziness and Panic Disorder."[12] In it, the authors summarized over thirty studies linking inner ear dysfunction with acute mental distress. "Some cases of panic disorder," they explained, "are triggered by misinterpreted stimuli from vestibular dysfunction that are interpreted as signifying imminent physical danger." The authors proposed that mistimed inner ear signals can set off a false alarm in a part of the brain called the locus coeruleus, which is the hair-trigger switch that trips in response to acute stress. It is in that part of the brain where adrenaline is manufactured and stored, just waiting to be released. It could be, surmised the team, that some people have a low threshold to release their bottled-up adrenaline; all it takes is an overexcited inner ear to discharge the load. For some, a little VR is enough to set things in motion.

The Harvard study, and others like it, offer circumstantial evidence that VR can spark psychological distress via the inner ear.[13] But these studies did not assess VR directly. In 2006, a research team at the University of Montreal did just that.[14] Their results confirmed that the anecdotal reports of post-VR symptoms were scientifically reproducible. In their study, led by psychologist Frederick Aardema, the Canadian team found that after twenty-five minutes in a virtual environment there was an increase in DP/DR symptoms and a diminished sense of presence in objective reality among a group of otherwise healthy subjects. Moreover, the higher the baseline DP/DR scores, the more likely VR was to trigger the dissociative symptoms. Importantly, Aardema did not find cases of outright panic among these healthy participants, but his results suggest that in a vulnerable person, VR might be enough to flip the switch. "While the magnitude of these effects are unclear and may last for only a short duration after exposure to VR," he writes, "it would be wise to take those results into consideration when using VR immersion with people who have preexisting clinical levels of dissociation."

For Gloria, there was a perfect storm of factors conspiring to trigger VR panic. First, we did not perform baseline testing for DP/DR susceptibility. Given her history of anxiety and PTSD, it's likely that Gloria would have scored higher than average. Aardema's research shows that such results are a risk factor for VR panic. Second, Gloria had never before been in VR. Because she did not have previous experience with VR, she had no way to acclimate to the physical effects of virtual immersion on the inner ear. Third, *Bear Blast* requires constant head movement and creates a sense of forward propulsion, which is sure to prompt inner ear turbulence. In contrast, the Cirque du Soleil app is a stationary experience.

But there's certainly more to it than that. For Gloria, the game summoned feelings of violence, adding a layer of emotional vulnerability. Somehow, combining *Bear Blast* with her history of abuse, anxiety, and PTSD formed a combustible mixture that triggered a panic attack. Scrambling the inner ear may have hastened Gloria's distress, but it cannot fully explain how knocking over bears could provoke such an explosive reaction. After all, the Cirque du Soleil app generated a different reaction, not only because it was less likely to cause cybersickness by virtue of limited head motion, but more so because it felt peaceful and familiar to Gloria. Something else happened in *Bear Blast*, and that something else is, to me at least, still a mystery.

As a consciousness-altering treatment, VR has effects on mind and body that are explainable to a point but that still escape a deterministic account. Unlike the cause-and-effect field of pharmacology, where scientists can point to which receptor or enzyme a drug activates or inhibits, VR therapies don't plug into a narrow receptor or flip a specific switch. Explaining the mechanism of a treatment that alters sensations, emotions, and cognitions is far more complicated. Notwithstanding the theory of embodied cognitions covered in Chapter 1, which offers a framework to help explain VR's effects on mind and body, all the science in the world cannot, as of yet, entirely explain why Gloria had a panic attack. Her story highlights what is arguably the most general potential risk of VR, namely, that therapies trafficking on subjective experience are difficult to standardize and control because perception varies so markedly from person to person.

Although I have tried throughout this book to support the science of immersive therapeutics using evidence and theories, the field remains nascent and is evolving; there's still so much to learn. While Gloria's story shows how VR pushes on certain pressure points in the body, like the vestibular system and locus coeruleus, it also highlights the explanatory limits of existing theories and reminds us that until we fully understand consciousness, we won't fully understand VR.

Ever since Gloria's episode I have been more cognizant about the potential of harm with VR and more mindful about screening for risk factors in other vulnerable patients.

VR can also have strong effects on children. I learned that lesson the hard way. At my son's school. I once set up a science fair VR demo and invited kids to experience the magic of immersive technology. I shared some low-key experiences, like lying on a beach and swimming with sea creatures, but I also brought the ledge jumper—the same experience I described at the beginning of this book—for the more adventurous students. I was a little nervous about letting kids jump off a virtual building, so I did what any father would do: experiment with my ten-year-old son. He affixed the goggles, went up the side of the building, and fearlessly jumped off without a moment of hesitation. No problem. A complete success.

Next, I tried it with a few of his friends. Same thing. They all loved it, one by one, and nobody showed even a hint of the existential fear that gripped my brain during the same freefall. Word quickly spread about the virtual leap. Before long, a line of children was queued up and ready to go. I must have put fifty kids through the experience without observing an adverse event. Before each child donned the headset I was careful to discuss what would happen. I also screened out kids who were afraid of heights or those who seemed too young to handle the experience. I obtained consent from parents before starting. I monitored them carefully as they went through the experience. All was fine.

It was somewhere around the fifty-first child when things went awry. He ascended the building and started to shake, first subtly, then more visibly.

"Hey, buddy," I said, "we should stop right here. I think we ought to take off the goggles."

"No, I'm fine. I want to do it."

"Okay, but it looks like you're getting a little shaky. We ought to call it a day here. No biggie."

"No, I'm okay, I want to keep going up."

I naively let him continue. And then, surrounded by his peers, his parents, and what seemed like a stadium full of spectators, a dark streak cut across his khaki pants, first pooling along his thigh, then navigating around his knee, and finally making a beeline for his ankles, where a stream of urine emerged into a rapidly expanding puddle around his feet on the gym floor.

End of demo. I wanted to disappear.

It turns out he was okay. I checked in with the boy and his parents after the incident. He seemed fine and the parents were understanding. But deep down, I worried he might not soon forget the indelible fear of scaling the building, however virtual, and the embarrassment of his visceral response.

The story of the science fair fiasco again emphasizes that overriding the brain is not an unmitigated good. Children, in particular, can be easily frightened while in VR. It is critical to take precautions whenever exposing young patients to immersive therapeutics.

Beyond fright, children can also develop false memories from VR. Whereas adults are able to distinguish fantasy from reality, children may confuse the two, especially when the virtual worlds seem so real. In one study by Stanford psychologists Kathryn Segovia and Jeremy Bailenson, titled "Virtually True," young children were divided into groups: some experienced swimming with orcas in VR, while others were simply asked to imagine swimming with whales.[15] The VR group got split up further: some children watched other kids swimming with the orcas, while others experienced a virtual doppelgänger of themselves swimming with the sea creatures. Then, the researchers checked back five days later to record what the kids remembered.

The results were striking: the children in VR were more likely to believe their virtual experience was truly real. And among those in the VR group, the children who saw their own self swimming were even more likely to recall the experience as an actual event. The very sense of virtual embodiment that convinced me I had a near-death experience in Mel Slater's lab was the same sense that instilled false memories in the Stanford pediatric study. As I sit here today, I know that I didn't *actually* depart my physical body while in VR; it just felt that way. But for young children, swimming with whales can become a bona fide experience, indistinguishable from any other real event. In their study, Segovia and Bailenson found that risk of false memories was strongest in the youngest kids, who averaged around four to five years old, but the researchers also detected false memories in some six- and seven-year-old participants. Once children reach eight to ten years of age, they develop an ability to think more logically and are less vulnerable to false memories.* That's why I restricted the ledge jump to older kids at the science fair (although, as I

---

* When I discussed this research with Mel Slater, he emphasized that these "false memories" are not really false at all. They happened. Although the whales weren't real, the experience of the whales was very real. We'll explore the slippery distinction between real and virtual reality in Chapter 11.

learned, the age cutoffs are not absolute rules). By the time children are twelve years old, they develop a coherent view of the world and can reason more critically. For these older children, there is minimal risk of VR creating false memories. Of course, we never set out to falsify memories as an explicit goal of VR, but if inadvertent false memories are positive and affirming, then there's little harm done. On the other hand, if false memories are negative, then clearly there could be harm.

Segovia and Bailenson's research offers a caveat to pediatric virtualists: take special care when using VR with young kids. Kate Donovan knows this well. As the clinical director of immersive technologies at Boston Children's Hospital, Donovan runs one of the largest pediatric VR programs in the world. Her team uses VR for everything from reducing pain from needle sticks to educating patients and their families about invasive procedures. "I am such an advocate for VR," she told me. "I don't want to overemphasize the negative things about VR, because honestly, if I had my way, I would put it in the hands of most all of my patients. But we still have to understand the safety of VR."

There are other unexpected consequences when using VR with children. Molly Easterlin, a pediatrician at Cedars-Sinai studying VR for children with inflammatory bowel disease, discovered that some parents had concerns nobody saw coming. Easterlin thought it would be a good idea to use VR while her patients were receiving intravenous medication, which can take upward of an hour while sitting in a chair. The procedure is boring and uncomfortable, so VR seemed like an ideal solution to pass the time and distract from pain. Not surprisingly, it helped a lot. The children reported less discomfort, anxiety, and boredom with VR. But a few parents worried that VR was artificially shielding their children from the adversity of the experience. "They didn't want their kids to suffer unnecessarily," Easterlin told me, "but they also felt like going through the procedure would help build character, sort of make their kids stronger. Some parents thought VR was a disservice. It was like VR took away an important and necessary part of their identity as a patient."

Personally, I can respect this parental point of view but remain agnostic about whether VR softens kids. Every child and every illness is different. But I know this much for sure: I've never heard anyone say that watching *SpongeBob SquarePants* or *Looney Toons* on TV might weaken kids' resolve to fight their illness. This concern—that VR is so powerful it can rob patients of the paradoxical silver lining of *being* a patient— speaks to what makes VR different from any other audiovisual platform ever created.

It would be unwise to ignore the ways VR makes it easier for kids to be patients. Research shows that VR can help children get through needle sticks, spinal taps, cast removals, dental procedures, and realignment of dislocated joints or bone fractures.[16] The technology is also helping children manage autism spectrum disorders, phobias, depression, anxiety, and neurological conditions.[17] The results of these studies, more than a hundred of them, are consistently positive. But it is the individual patient stories—not the numerical results of meta-analyses—that are so moving and compelling. For example, at the University of Michigan, children receiving chemotherapy ride a virtual roller coaster or accompany the beloved U of M football players as they enter the stadium, all to distract their mind from illness.[18] A boy sidelined by blood clots at Cedars-Sinai enters a fantastical, immersive playland to gain respite from the constant pain, beeping machines, and needle sticks in the hospital.[19] At Stanford University, children preparing for surgery play with Sevo the Dragon, an interactive VR character that transforms anesthesia into an adventure.[20] At the City University of Hong Kong, children with autism are using VR to learn new emotional and social skills.[21] And at the University Medical Center Amsterdam, children with cerebral palsy learn how to strengthen their gait by following cartoon avatars in a virtual environment.[22] These examples, and many others, demonstrate the inspiring potential of VR to help some of our most vulnerable patients. There are risks of using VR with children, but there are also profound benefits. We need to strike a balance.

While doctors await additional evidence about optimizing the safety of pediatric VR, Kate Donovan recommends a commonsense approach when using immersive therapeutics for kids. She advises limiting VR sessions to no more than twenty minutes at a time, if that, and she endorses taking at least a thirty-minute break between sessions. These guidelines are especially important for the youngest kids at risk of false memories. Donovan advocates using software that avoids stressful adventures in favor of pleasant experiences that promote self-efficacy and happiness. She also suggests coupling VR treatment with support from child life specialists working with patients and their families. By combining socially responsible VR with the human touch of pediatric care, immersive therapeutics have great potential to ease pain, calm nerves, and improve health in children suffering from acute and chronic diseases.

Using immersive therapeutics in kids raises the specter of another concern that we haven't yet discussed: screen time. We have all heard about the harmful effects of prolonged screen time. Isn't VR just screen time turned up to 11? Can't patients—both children and adults—become dependent on VR screens, just as they can with opioids? Will patients who use VR risk disappearing into virtual fantasies rather than facing reality?

Although I included hundreds of references in the back of this book, none of them address the addictive potential of therapeutic VR because the literature is scant. In contrast, there is a vast literature on the risks of video games and smart devices that is extensively reviewed elsewhere and beyond the scope of this discussion.[23] But in healthcare, where the goal is to treat disease and alleviate suffering—not merely to entertain—the research on VR addiction is lacking.

There's a scientific aphorism to bear in mind here: "Absence of evidence is not evidence of absence." In other words, just because the literature is scant does not confirm that therapeutic VR is without risk. So, in the absence of evidence, I've had to collect my own evidence.

Our team is always on the lookout for signs of VR dependency. We routinely monitor how long patients spend living in virtual worlds, and, so far at least, we have not detected signs of abuse. Patients in our trials average around fifteen to twenty minutes per day in VR, and almost never more than an hour. We typically record a steep drop-off after four weeks of use. Many people tire of VR, or get bored of it, or just don't want to spend much time in VR due to the risk of cybersickness. That's okay, so long as VR offered a benefit and allowed patients to learn something new and valuable, or to improve their lives in real reality. Our goal is not for people to be in VR forever. The goal is to train the mind to appreciate real reality, and to have a healthier mind-set upon reemerging into the world. When we check back months later, very few of our patients are still using VR on a daily basis, much less at all; they've graduated from treatment and are back living their lives.

There are rare exceptions. One time we detected a patient who was using VR every few hours. His use was so frequent that it seemed like an error. A research associate called to inquire. The patient said that swimming with dolphins kept him off opioids, so he used the headset whenever he could. VR was staving off a worse fate than overexposure to marine life. Although we don't encourage patients to stay in VR quite that often, we considered this trade-off to be clinically acceptable. But he was an outlier.

I asked other VR experts to share their own views. Skip Rizzo, whom we met back in Chapter 2, has worked in therapeutic VR for nearly thirty years and agrees that VR addiction is rare in healthcare. "We just don't see it," he told me. "I understand why people are concerned, just like people were concerned when moving pictures came out in the early 1900s, or when *Pac-Man* came out. I don't want to make light of it, and we're always watching carefully. But VR addiction is not something we see when our patients use VR for health reasons."

Jeremy Bailenson at Stanford, whose research we discussed earlier in this chapter, also agrees. "There is a sense from many people that VR is sinister—that it represents the nail in the coffin of a natural, social-oriented mode of human life that has been gradually dying away," he writes. "I think this view seriously underestimates real life."[24] Bailenson emphasizes that VR can't come close to simulating every granular detail of reality and, "in a strange way, VR helps you to appreciate the real world more."

This core idea—that virtual reality strengthens our appreciation of real reality—dates back to the earliest days of VR. Jaron Lanier, who you'll recall coined the term "virtual reality," discovered this perception-boosting power while originally developing the technology. "Once your nervous system adapts to a virtual world and then you come back, you have a chance to experience being born again in microcosm. The most ordinary surface, cheap wood or plain dirt, is bejeweled in infinite detail for a short while. To look into another's eyes is almost too intense."[25] Lanier concluded that living in a simulated reality, even for a short time, cultivates a sense of awe and wonder about the real world. "As VR progresses in the future," he predicted, "human perception will be nurtured by it and will learn to find ever more depth in physical reality."

But as VR progresses we must still learn how to optimize its benefits and limit its risks. Virtualists will benefit from guidance on how to balance the pros and cons of VR and how to communicate that balance to patients and their families. This insight came into focus for me while visiting, of all places, a major motion picture studio. It was there that I realized VR mandates its own unique form of oversight.

Sony Picture Studios is a sprawling campus in Culver City, California, that houses the corporation's motion picture, television, and music divisions. In the beating heart of the complex, just a stone's throw from the *Wheel of Fortune* and *Shark Tank* sets, lies a large, windowless building labeled Stage 7. Inside the transformed sound stage is a cutting-edge research and development facility established by Sony in 2018 to leverage technologies throughout its multinational divisions. The skunkworks project, called Innovation Studios, was established to develop and implement novel technologies that serve common interests across organizational silos. Selling millions of PlayStation VR headsets around the world, Sony is among the leaders in promoting immersive entertainment. Among its remits, Innovation Studios is advancing the science of immersive optics to create new ways of delighting audiences.[26]

It is next to Stage 7, at the studio commissary, where I met Scot Barbour, then vice president of production for Innovation Studios, to discuss VR. A quick-witted technophile with decades of experience building and testing innovations, Barbour knows a lot about the technical features of VR—way more than I do. But there's something he hasn't yet solved.

"We need better guidance around managing the risks of VR," he told me. Barbour explained that designing for VR is not like designing a 2-D game, producing a TV show, or creating a movie. VR introduces new issues that entertainment producers never had to consider before. Those issues are not just about the complexity of designing 360-degree immersive scenes. No, Barbour was talking about something different. He was talking about the complexity of designing around the psychology of a VR user.

"We already have rating systems for video games and movies. But what's appropriate in traditional media may not work in VR," he said. For example, Barbour explained that watching *The Smurfs* on TV might seem totally benign, but the same scene in 2-D can become terrifying in immersive 3-D if a child finds herself playing with the Smurfs on the side of a cliff or atop a high mountain.

In VR, it's not enough to just tell a good story; software designers must also consider how the user physically experiences the story. When Papa Smurf is telling a campfire story on TV, nobody bats an eyelash. But when a child is sitting right next to that blazing campfire, he might become anxious and want to escape, no matter what Papa Smurf is talking about. That child might not be having fun at all. Unlike passively watching a movie or a TV show, where the viewer is just a spectator, being embedded in a scene convinces the mind that it's literally part of the action. Personal space matters in virtual life just as it does in real life. And that's Barbour's point: VR has consequences like no other media.

James Spiegel, the VR bioethicist we met earlier in this chapter, agrees with Barbour that VR can have unexpected negative consequences. The "Faustian bargain" of using VR, as Spiegel calls it, requires guardrails to protect against misuse. "Industry leaders would be wise," he writes, "to caution potential users more earnestly and aggressively, even if this results in slightly lower sales, by enlisting game rating agencies to classify their products or perhaps by creating their own industry rating board like the MPAA for the film industry. Even aside from public interest in users' psychological and even physical safety, the aim of mitigating potential legal problems would recommend such a move."[27]

So far, Spiegel and Barbour's request hasn't been met. The major game-rating organizations have not yet developed unique criteria for classifying VR programs. Instead, consumer VR games are rated like traditional 2-D games; the focus of ratings is on content, not on the physical embodiment of the content—the characteristic of physical embodiment remains murky and challenging to measure. For now, VR companies must settle with posting disclaimers and warnings in boilerplate legalese.

In the meantime, for those of us using VR in healthcare, it is crucial to establish a code of conduct that limits patients from harm, wherever possible. In 2016, two philosophy professors from the University of Mainz, Michael Madary and Thomas Metzinger, answered the call for an ethical framework.[28] In their treatise, published in the journal *Frontiers in Robotics and AI*, the philosophers identified a list of principles governing the ethics of VR. For me, three of their precepts stand out as most relevant to healthcare:

1. *Non-maleficence.* Although there will always be some inherent risk with VR, using the technology with a patient is acceptable when the perceived benefits outweigh the potential risks. However, Madary and Metzinger entreat that "no experiment should be conducted using virtual reality with the foreseeable consequence that it will cause serious or lasting harm to a subject."

2. *Informed consent.* Anyone offered therapeutic VR should receive a clear explanation that the treatment might cause side effects, and that not all adverse events are known.

3. *Transparency.* Here, Madary and Metzinger worry that technophiles and entrepreneurs may overhype the benefits of therapeutic VR beyond what the research shows. They urge stakeholders to be forthright about the limits and potential risks of VR. They also encourage developers to partner with healthcare professionals when building therapeutic products. "VR researchers aiming at new clinical applications," they write, "should therefore work slowly and carefully, in close collaboration with physicians who may be better

situated to make informed judgments about the suitability of particular patients for new trials."

Although Madary and Metzinger's code of ethics is not binding, it offers a blueprint for others to follow. "Its publication," writes journalist Daniel Oberhaus, "marks an important first step toward ensuring that the proliferation of virtual reality technology doesn't lead us into some *Matrix*-esque hell."[29] That may be too stark an assessment, but as a doctor trained in the ethos of primum non nocere, I do find Madary and Metzinger's cautionary plea for transparency to be compelling. I sometimes worry that my own enthusiasm for therapeutic VR could be misconstrued as unfettered proselytizing. I am enthusiastic about VR and I've seen it do good. That's why I wrote this book. But as a scientist, I want to know about the good and the bad. I want to understand the risks of VR and be transparent about them. I want to help my patients with mind-body technologies, but I also must do my best to protect them from unintended consequences.

We may never achieve the ideal of primum non nocere with therapeutic VR, but we sure can try.

CHAPTER NINE

The VR Pharmacy

I'M DREAMING WITH MY EYES WIDE OPEN. AT LEAST, THAT'S HOW IT feels as I fly with a flock of birds through a tunnel of flowers stretched across a pastel sky. Down below are giant Chinese lanterns, each surrounded by a ring of spotlights cutting through misty air. Up ahead is, well, it's hard to say. There's some kind of illuminated cavern opening itself to me. In the middle of the cavern is a human form with massive fronds sprouting from its head. The details come into view as I enter this vacuous space. Now I see the giant metallic torso of a woman with glowing cheekbones and neon green streaks flowing off her head into the ceiling. Trees are sprouting behind her from a floor filled with colorful polygons. I hear gorgeous orchestral music.

Then I notice something totally unexpected. My family is here. I am surrounded by glowing orbs, and within each orb is a picture of a family member. There's my daughter. And there's my son. There goes my wife. And there's Pacha, our beloved golden retriever. I'm literally surrounded by my family in this ethereal place. It sounds corny, but my heart is filled with love.

I have just experienced *TRIPP*, an aptly named VR program that serves up a menu of trippy therapeutic worlds. When you "tripp," as the developers call using their program, you first select a desired mood that best fits your immediate needs. Want to chill out? *TRIPP* can help. Need to get out of a funk? *TRIPP* can pump you up. Nanea Reeves, CEO of *TRIPP*, calls her program the world's first "adaptive digiceutical."

And that's the key: it is truly adaptive. *TRIPP* customizes its virtual worlds around each user. Incorporating family photos is just the start. The team also composed adaptive music that creates a personalized soundscape designed to trigger specific moods. *TRIPP* uses a technique called binaural beats, which means the left and right ear register tones at slightly different frequencies. Research shows that by varying the sound frequency between ears, composers can manipulate brain waves— those synchronized electrical currents that arise from communicating neurons—to a desired frequency.[1] For example, when the difference in sound frequency between ears is set at 10 hertz, the brain flips into an *alpha pattern*, which encourages relaxation. When the difference is set between 14 and 100 hertz, also called a *beta pattern*, the result is enhanced concentration and alertness. Dial the difference down to only 4 hertz and a *theta pattern* emerges, which promotes meditation and creativity. By exploiting the brain's response to binaural beats, *TRIPP* combines the power of VR and music to shape emotions. "We built a mood-on-demand platform powered by VR," says Reeves. "We're taking proven techniques of mindful meditation and sound therapy, and then amplifying them with the power of immersive VR."

As I reflect on my experience in *TRIPP*, I'm especially struck by the impact of seeing my family in that virtual world. The result was the same mystical feeling I experienced in Slater's out-of-body machine or Sackman's meditative breathing app, but this time, rather than experiencing a generic world, I was surrounded by a space personally adapted to me.

If VR is a therapy, then we need a VR pharmacy. As a doctor, I need shelves full of VR treatments that are safe, effective, and that I can personalize for each individual patient, just like *TRIPP* was personalized to me. That is, after all, how I use drug therapy: I consider each patient's unique health profile, discuss goals of treatment, and then prescribe a tailored drug regimen designed to improve quality of life. I wouldn't be a very effective doctor if I gave everyone the same prescription, and I wouldn't be a very good virtualist if I gave everyone the same VR treatment.

In order to craft a personalized treatment plan, I need to think about the *three rights*: selecting the *right* immersive therapeutic, for the *right* patient, and using it at the *right* time.

By the "right therapeutic," I mean selecting a treatment that addresses individual patient needs, is evidence-based, is proven to work in the appropriate clinical setting, and is safe. The right program should also employ a mechanism of action, or MOA in the parlance of doctors, that counteracts the targeted disease. Just like with medical therapy, where I consider the MOA of a drug when selecting treatments for a patient, I also need to consider the MOA of an immersive therapy when personalizing VR treatments. If the target condition is pain, for example, then I need to dampen inner pain signals through inattentional blindness, time contraction, and gate control theory. If the target is anxiety, then I need to promote a cognitive flow state. If I'm treating dementia or schizophrenia, then I need to strengthen self-identity. If I am managing obesity or anorexia, then I need to enhance healthy body attention. The four MOAs of immersion offer a framework for how to organize the VR pharmacy; it's how I think about selecting the right virtual treatment.

But even people with the exact same condition may benefit from different VR programs. Take two patients with acute pain from, say, a bone fracture. Both patients might benefit from VR distraction therapy, yet each might have a unique preference for the type of distraction. One might prefer to lie on a beach while the other might prefer a forest. Or maybe one patient likes to swim with dolphins while the other enjoys floating through a fantasy landscape, like I did in *TRIPP*. In all of these cases, the MOA is to dampen pain signals through inattentional blindness via distraction. But if we had a way to individualize treatments, then maybe we could do better than a one-size-fits-all approach.

A simple way to tailor treatment is to ask patients what they prefer. When I approach people with a library of immersive therapeutics, I typically describe the options and ask what they want to try. That's easy enough. In Chapter 4 we learned how Alexandre Dumais uses a similar approach when personalizing virtual avatars for his patients with schizophrenia. Through trial and error, he constructs a face and voice that best depicts each patient's unique hallucination. If the avatar isn't quite right, then Dumais goes back to the drawing board and makes updates until his patient perceives it to be realistic.

But I think we can do even better. Consider again how I select VR treatments for pain. I describe what we have in the VR library and ask people to choose. But not every patient can predict what will work best. Many have never experienced VR, so preselecting a virtual environment can be challenging. Others are familiar with VR, yet they haven't mulled over what type of distraction works best for their pain. Still others may have so many preferences that they have difficulty deciding among the options. Having too many choices is not a problem when there's ample time to explore the entire VR library. But in some cases there is little time to experiment. Think about someone about to receive a spinal tap in the emergency department; a trial-and-error approach is not feasible because there's only one chance to select the right experience. If there were a more sophisticated and efficient technique for pinpointing the right program for each patient, then maybe we could optimize clinical outcomes.

One technique for customizing treatment involves a short computer-administered questionnaire and a bit of math. Our research team uses a technique called conjoint analysis, which is a quantitative method to elucidate patient preferences. The technique first originated at The Wharton School, the famed school of business at the University of Pennsylvania, to help product managers understand consumer preferences. For example, imagine a consumer in the market for a new laptop computer. Different computers have different attributes that may impact the consumer's decision. These attributes include such things as price, storage capacity, screen size, processing speed, durability, and weight. Computer manufacturers like Apple or Microsoft want to know how consumers will navigate these attributes when selecting a laptop. So they perform market research using conjoint analysis to precisely quantify preferences. In a typical exercise, a consumer evaluates a pair of product descriptions side by side, each with a unique combination of attributes, and selects one perceived to be better. Next, the respondent views another comparison and again selects the preferred profile. The analysis software continues to draw up new comparisons that become increasingly difficult for the respondent to distinguish. Before long, the software computes each consumer's likes and dislikes. After surveying hundreds or thousands of prospective buyers and analyzing the data, companies can build products that meet their customers' needs.

Although conjoint analysis was originally designed to optimize product development, the technique is now used in healthcare to assess patient preferences.[2] For example, our team built a free app called *IBD&me* that helps people with inflammatory bowel disease (IBD) navigate among competing medical therapies.[3] Just like consumer products have different attributes, so do medicines. Patients need to consider out-of-pocket expenses, risk of serious side effects, likelihood of short-term relief, long-term remission rates, and mode of administration when selecting a medicine. *IBD&me* employs conjoint analysis to generate a personalized report depicting what each patient values in selecting the best medicine. Our research found that virtually no two patients share the exact same preferences, meaning that selecting the right treatment requires nuance; a one-size-fits-all approach falls short.[4]

The same assessment approach can work for tailoring VR treatments. Rather than asking patients if they like the beach or a forest or a desert scene, a computer program can systematically pose the questions. Using conjoint analysis, patients can view a set of photos or short videos that depict immersive environments. As patients make their choices, the software zeros in on helping the patient select the right environment through a series of increasingly specific choices. Not only can it optimize the visual scene (want a stream through your forest?), but it can also customize the music, control the amount of exploration (want to stay still or go on a journey?), tailor color schemes, and personalize the degree of interactivity

(want to just watch, or do you prefer a meditative breathing exercise?).
Conjoint analyses can be further modified by the medical indication. For
example, someone receiving a spinal tap cannot roll over, much less move
their head ninety degrees without disrupting the procedure. In that instance, the virtual environment should be entirely forward-facing. Same
thing for people with a very stiff neck, or patients undergoing dental
work—it could be harmful to include 360-degree images in these scenarios. When efficiently administered on a bedside tablet device or clinic
computer, conjoint analysis has the potential to enhance outcomes by personalizing and optimizing immersive therapeutics.

The second "right" for virtualists is selecting the "right patient" for a
VR treatment. The options for children in pain, for example, may be different than the options for women in labor. In both cases, the desired
MOA is to dampen inner pain signals. But delivering that MOA requires
different techniques because these are different types of patients. At
Stanford University, Tom Caruso, a pediatric anesthesiologist, uses a virtual fishing game called *Bait* to distract kids from their pain. At Cedars-
Sinai, Melissa Wong, a high-risk obstetrician, uses a Lamaze-style VR
breathing app to guide her patients through labor and delivery.[5] Both
doctors are trying to relieve pain by dampening inner pain signals, but
the method varies markedly between kids and laboring women.

We also need to think about susceptibility to risks. Think back to
Gloria's story in Chapter 8. Could we have predicted that Gloria would
have a panic attack after playing *Bear Blast* in the hospital? Maybe. Her
story indicates that we should evaluate for side effects prior to using VR.
If we had measured her risk of depersonalization and derealization, or
DP/DR, which we examined in Chapter 8, then we might have predicted
the adverse reaction. Yet, at the same time, Gloria reveled in being on the
Cirque du Soleil stage, proving that it wasn't VR, per se, that caused her
panic—it was the software *program* that triggered her existential crisis.
We just picked the wrong VR treatment.

Gloria's story reveals that a VR headset is like a syringe—both are
merely devices that deliver a therapy. The device itself is unimportant;

it's what passes *through* the device that matters. For a syringe, it's about what medicine is injected. For an immersive therapeutic, it's about what the patient sees, feels, hears, and experiences as she enters a virtual world. Therapeutic VR is not about the headset itself, particularly because headsets are constantly modernizing, but about what software is pumped through that headset.

As virtualists become more sophisticated at selecting the right treatment for the right patient, they will need to consider a range of parameters. Not all patients achieve the same benefits from the same VR therapy, because everyone is different. There are many factors that predict whether or not a patient will benefit from a particular VR therapy, ranging from clinical variables to demographic characteristics to psychosocial attributes. Because some of these factors are more predictive than others, virtualists need to determine how best to weigh each one in their decision-making. This can be done by instinct, but math can help, too.

In other areas of medicine, doctors use a statistical technique called regression analysis to fine-tune treatment decisions. The idea of regression analysis is to consider multiple factors, mathematically weigh the importance of each factor, and then crunch the numbers to yield an accurate prediction of a clinically important outcome. For example, doctors determine who is next in line for a liver transplant by running a regression analysis on everyone in the queue, and then rank-ordering patients based on their risk of imminent death (thus justifying who should get the next available liver). Regression analyses are also used to predict who should get certain types of chemotherapy, or who is at risk for a heart attack, and so forth. There are thousands of algorithms that patients and their doctors can use to optimize decisions. Some are more accurate than others, but the good algorithms are useful tools that support shared decision-making between doctors and their patients.

Therapeutic VR will benefit from the same type of precision. That's why our research team is testing algorithms to hone patient selection. So far, we've focused on predicting which patients with pain will benefit most from VR. Our results indicate that several factors can help spot patients most likely to benefit.

One of the most important factors is pain intensity. Patients with pain scores greater than 7 out of 10 points—a high level of pain—experience the greatest benefits from VR. In our research at Cedars-Sinai, patients with high pain intensity reported a 3-point drop in pain immediately after a VR treatment compared to a 1-point drop for those with less pain.[6] In both groups the effect was statistically significant, but the benefit was larger in the group experiencing more intense pain.

This difference is not because people with high pain scores have numerically farther to drop on the scale, but rather it has more to do with the nature of severe pain versus moderate pain. People with severe pain not only experience a high physical intensity of pain, but they also may endure a high emotional impact from pain. We cannot always prevent physical pain, but with the right medicine we can address emotional pain. "Pain is inevitable," said the Buddha, "but suffering is optional." VR modifies both sensory *and* emotional pain, as we learned in Chapter 3, which may explain why VR has a relatively larger effect for people with high amounts of pain. Recall the research on VR for burn victims and women in labor. In both cases, VR not only reduced the physical intensity of extreme pain, but it also caused patients to spend less time ruminating about their pain and to have less anxiety from their pain. VR can do this for people with moderate pain, too, but its dual benefits appear to help those with severe pain even more.

Age also matters. We've discovered that VR is more effective in older than younger people with pain. For every increased decade of age there is an additional 0.6 point reduction in pain from VR. We don't know for sure why this is, but one possibility is the existence of a "digital divide" that separates people who grew up with digital technologies like the internet and smartphones, and those who didn't. Younger patients often have higher expectations of technology and may require more sophisticated simulations to feel moved.

I remember one day, in particular, when I was consulted by a colleague to treat a couple of his patients with VR. One was an elderly man suffering from intense cancer pain. He opted to relax on a beach. He couldn't believe what he was seeing.

"Where am I?" he asked.

"Well, you're on a beach in Hawaii."

"How? How'd I get here? How did this happen?"

"It's only pictures of a beach. You're still here with us in the hospital, but the pictures make you feel like you're on a beach."

"This is magic," he said.

When we took him out of VR, he seemed utterly perplexed by the transition. The effect was so intense that I'm not sure whether he felt literally transported to Hawaii, as if he'd been beamed there and back, Star Trek style. I've seen this happen many times over, where people struggle to square the physics of being in two realities at once.

Yet, later that same morning, I used VR with a twenty-year-old man recovering from an ankle fracture. He had used VR before and was very familiar with the technology, but he was still willing to give it a try. I put him on the same beach as the elderly patient, but this young man was nonplussed.

"Uh, this is cool. But do you have anything else I can try?"

We put him on the helicopter tour over Iceland. Same response. A touch of curiosity, maybe, but nothing special.

"Do you have any games?"

We tried *Bear Blast*, the game Gloria used that triggered a panic attack. Again, not impressed.

"Can I skydive in this? Or surf? I'm into extreme sports."

Our VR library didn't have what he needed. Compared to the elderly patient, VR didn't make as much of a difference in the younger patient because he was familiar with VR. As a digital native, the younger patient had expectations about what the technology could deliver. This doesn't mean that young people cannot benefit from therapeutic VR, because they can and do, but it does mean that virtualists need to consider age when selecting the right program for the right patient.

There are many other factors to consider, like the type of pain, location of pain, frequency of pain, and so forth. Demographic characteristics may also be important to load into an algorithm, like a patient's gender, race, or ethnicity. Clinical factors, such as baseline anxiety or depression, number of medical conditions, or overall morbidity, are also likely to predict VR treatment response. In short, optimizing patient selection is not a unidimensional problem; selecting the right VR treatment for the right patient requires a more sophisticated approach than simple trial and error or educated guesses.

So far, we've talked about the first two "rights" of personalizing VR therapy—giving the *right* VR treatment to the *right* patient. Then there's the third right, which is giving that treatment at the *right time*. Here I mean that virtualists must consider how best to dose VR, just like when doctors administer drugs at a prescribed frequency (e.g., "take twice daily") and for a discrete period of time (e.g., "take for fourteen days").

How often and for how long should patients use VR? VR dosing depends on why it's being prescribed in the first place. In our pain research, for example, we generally recommend using VR for about ten to fifteen minutes at a time, three times per day, and as needed for a pain breakthrough. We also instruct our patients not to use VR for more than twenty minutes at a time, and always to take a thirty-minute break between sessions.

There's also nuance around when best to dose VR treatments as pain cycles up and down; the optimal timing can vary from person to person. Consider Tom Norris, a patient who uses VR to manage chronic pain. Norris, a retired lieutenant colonel of the US Air Force, knows how to get through tough times. He uses VR alongside a range of medical and mind-body treatments to keep ahead of his daily aches and pains. "The VR really helps," he told me. "But I've got to say, when the pain gets out of control and hits 11 out of 10, it's too late for VR. It can't touch that kind of pain." Instead, Norris uses VR while the pain is building but before it peaks; that's the best time for him to derail pain signals before he has to reach for his meds.

All of these examples indicate that there's an art and science to prescribing VR therapy. Just like with medical therapy, virtualists need to evaluate the whole clinical picture, consider the evidence for individual VR treatment options, and do their level best to match the right treatment, for the right patient, at the right time.

When all three "rights" align, I call the result precision immersion. This term is inspired by the more general notion of precision medicine that has become popular over the last decade. Precision medicine, as defined by the National Institutes of Health (NIH), is an approach that will "allow doctors and researchers to predict more accurately which treatment and prevention strategies for a particular disease will work in which groups of people." The NIH further explains that "it is in contrast to a one-size-fits-all approach, in which disease treatment and prevention strategies are developed for the average person, with less consideration for the differences between individuals."[7] Precision immersion therapy puts the patient in the center. It seeks to understand the biopsychosocial profile of an individual patient, and, when successful, offers tools to help doctors select the right therapy from the VR pharmacy, prescribe it to the right patient, and dose it with the right frequency, the right duration, and the right timing.

When I think back to my time in *TRIPP*, I felt in the center of that therapeutic world—literally. I felt like the programmers had custom-built an environment around my personal needs. I was surrounded by my family, enriched by music that was acoustically programmed to nudge my brain for a specific purpose, and embedded in a world designed to achieve a mood that I had personally selected from a menu of options. It felt precise, and I think that's why it was so effective.

The personal touch matters, not only for pharmaceuticals, but also for digiceuticals. I learned that in *TRIPP*; but I also witnessed, at first hand, how fit-for-purpose VR not only improves physical and mental health but also can boost spiritual health.

For this part of the story we have to go to church.

Pastor Kelvin Sauls has an infectious smile and a playful laugh that makes anyone who meets him feel good inside. Sauls, the visionary former leader of Holman United Methodist Church in South Los Angeles, California, views his role not only as a spiritual advisor to a large African American congregation but also as a guardian of health for his parishioners and the surrounding community. Pastor Sauls had noticed that many people in his church were suffering from high blood pressure, and too many were having strokes and heart attacks at an early age. He vowed to do something about it.

"It's not good enough for me to save souls in the sanctuary and then serve food in the fellowship hall that's so unhealthy it kills the body," Sauls told me. "It is hypocritical of me to not be concerned about the whole being, body and soul."

Under Sauls's leadership, the Holman Church established a collaboration with Bernice Coleman, a scientist at Cedars-Sinai who specializes in cardiovascular medicine. Coleman and Sauls decided it was time to combine the expertise of an academic medical center with the grassroots, community-driven initiative of Holman Church to address a silent killer that disproportionately affects the African American community. The key, they decided, was to make it personal.

The collaboration led to the Sodium Healthy Living Project, also called So-HELP. This culturally tailored program, funded by the Hearst Foundation, teaches participants where salt is predominantly found in the African American diet, how to substitute offending foods with low-salt alternatives, and how salt can damage vital organs. Coleman's team created a twelve-week program to teach parishioners about high blood pressure and its health effects, focusing on the role of salt as a modifiable cause of hypertension. To supplement the program, our VR group created a virtual environment that allowed people to fly through their own heart, kidney, and blood vessels so as to experience, at first hand, the damaging effects of salt on their body. Then, after observing their organs up close and personal, the parishioners emerged from their virtual bodies into a virtual kitchen, where they learned how to introduce low-salt ingredients into their diet. Finally, they walked out onto a virtual beach where they experienced a virtual sermon from Pastor Sauls on the importance of healthy living. By combining the power of traditional education, immersive VR environments, and the personal touch of a spiritual leader, So-HELP conveyed lessons in a way that no trifold educational brochure or health video could ever accomplish.*

---

* You can watch clips of So-HELP at this website: www.virtualmedicine.health/So -HELP.

Pastor Sauls nicknamed the project VR-TIME, for Vitality Realized Together in Meaningful Engagement.[8] The secret ingredient, he explained, was directly engaging participants in their own care. "We came together to fashion a program that invites folk into interactive and experiential health education," said Sauls. "And once we got them right where we needed them, we slid in the technology. Before they knew it, they had stuff all up on their head and on their face listening to things, and then they were amazed that my voice was right up in there!"

Similar to *TRIPP*, where I was surrounded by my own family in a therapeutic environment, So-HELP surrounded parishioners with the presence and wisdom of their own spiritual leader. That personal engagement helped bring the material to life. What might otherwise have been a dry educational offering about the physiology of hypertension became a vibrant, immersive, individualized journey through mind, body, and soul.

But there was more to it than just pumping the voice of Pastor Sauls into a VR headset. The very content of the VR program, and the foundational curriculum delivered by Coleman, was developed in partnership with end users from the ground up. Not one line of code was programmed until the vision and scope of So-HELP had first been cocreated with the parishioners and had been aligned with their expressed needs and preferences. This was about precision immersion.

"If you're a researcher," said Pastor Sauls, "don't design stuff for folk and expect to co-opt them into your program. You've got to work with them as partners. You've got to go on a journey together. That way, there's a sense of accountability built right in. When people participate in their own health, they're more likely to stick with the program."

Coleman and her team set out to create a culturally sensitive, custom-built educational program. They engaged with Sauls and his church leadership, assembled focus groups among the parishioners, and conducted interviews to understand preferences and unmet needs that VR might address. Coleman's team then worked with our group at Cedars-Sinai to develop storyboards for the VR program with input from participants. Every detail was carefully constructed in a collaborative partnership. Even the voice-over within the VR was selected with care;

the team auditioned over fifty voice actors before settling on one who was considered to be effective and culturally sensitive. It was only after months of work that we finally began to program the virtual environments and record the voice-overs.

VR was one part of the So-HELP intervention. Coleman also delivered interactive classes on diet, nutrition, cardiovascular physiology, and self-monitoring. The parishioners wore Fitbits to track their steps and sleep, and each received a blood pressure cuff to monitor their numbers from home. Nurses called the participants twice per week to check in, offer encouragement, and answer questions. This was a holistic intervention.

It was only after six weeks of Coleman's curriculum that we finally introduced VR. By then, the participants had already received education and were ready to reinforce what they had learned. "As a nurse," Coleman said, "I spend a lot of my time educating patients from a *'do you see what I'm saying?'* perspective. The beauty of VR is that I can literally show them what I'm saying. They can see it for themselves. It reinforces the learning."[9]

"VR can't take over the world by itself," cautioned Sauls. "We need to lay the groundwork with experiential learning. By the time we brought in VR the seeds had been planted, the soil had been tilled, and they were ready to go into that virtual world together."

Sauls and Coleman emphasize that technology is only part of the solution. And they're right. We learned the same lesson in our VR analgesia study I described in Chapter 7, where our first patient completely forgot about VR because he wasn't sufficiently engaged in the project. In that study, which used VR cognitive behavioral therapy to battle pain and lower opioid use, we assigned a "digital health coach" to check in on patients, similar to the So-HELP nursing model developed by Coleman.

"I love technology, don't get me wrong," Sauls told me. "I'm all about high tech. But that has to be accompanied by the personal touch. *By the Holy Touch.* It's not just about putting a screen in front of people. It's about inviting people into catalytic spaces so they can participate in meaningful engagement."

The results of So-HELP were encouraging. Fifty-six people completed the twelve-week program, and their systolic blood pressure dropped by an average of seven points over the course of the study.[10] That's significant, because research shows that even a three-point drop is enough to begin reducing the risks of high blood pressure. The pilot study was small and there was no control group, but Coleman detected an early signal that So-HELP could make a difference. Her team also observed lower stress and higher social support scores among the participants, suggesting the program improved overall biopsychosocial health, not just blood pressure.

"It was the individual stories," Sauls told me, "that really stood out." One man battling cancer joined the study and came every week, never missing a class or a VR treatment session. He always was the first to arrive and the last to leave. "Throughout his time in the study," Sauls recalled, "we could see a change in his attitude. A change in his physical appearance. A change in his eyes. Because through this experience he was able to engage in his health. I'll never forget when we brought in the VR. He had a blast applying what he learned through the health education sessions, and now he was actually able to *see* this stuff, hear the music, hear my voice. He wasn't engaging in escapism. He was engaging in a new way with his mind and body."

The man died about a year after participating in So-HELP. Pastor Sauls delivered his eulogy, which he titled "Fighting the Good Fight." Sauls recounted, "I believe that So-HELP gave him new resiliency and courage to fight the good fight. This brother didn't go down without a fight. We were privileged to be with him together 'til the last breath he took. Vitality realized together in meaningful engagement," Sauls said, repeating his mantra. "This was about VR-TIME."

The So-HELP study is a model for aligning the "three rights" of precision immersion. Recall that the first two "rights" are selecting the right treatment for the right patient. In the case of So-HELP, the program was precision-built to meet the needs of a specific group of people. It was designed with a targeted MOA to address a specific health issue. Using the four-mechanism framework introduced in Chapter 1 and reviewed earlier in this chapter, So-HELP has an MOA of enhancing healthy body attention regarding the corrosive effect of salt. The third "right" is about the timing and duration of treatment. Here, the VR treatment was not introduced until after six weeks of standardized education, self-monitoring, and health coaching. It was then continued for six additional weeks. So-HELP is a specific, targeted, and protocolized digiceutical.

As the shelves of the VR pharmacy continue to fill with treatments like So-HELP, virtualists will need a method to determine whether new immersive therapeutics are worth using in clinical practice. What makes the good ones worthwhile? How do we objectively judge the value of a new program, like So-HELP?

Having tried over one hundred different therapeutic VR programs, I can testify that some are better than others. I remember one treatment for chronic pain that felt like an Atari video game from the 1970s and 1980s. I put on the headset and saw the silhouette of a man facing me from about ten meters away. It looked like one of those targets on a firing range. Sure enough, I was instructed to begin shooting the silhouette in the part of its body where I experience pain. I occasionally get headaches around my eyes and was feeling a bit of a headache that day, so I decided to shoot this man's virtual eyes, although I didn't actually see any eyes, just a dark head. Then, a pixelated line flew out from my face and slowly made its way to the man, striking his face with a bang. There was even a little "shooting" noise, like a laser beam out of Star Wars or something. I kept shooting this man over and over, and then the treatment was over. I came out and the developers asked whether my headache was any better. Ummm . . . not quite.

That experience made me wonder how the developers decided to create that particular program. For me, it wasn't effective at all. I was unclear why it was even rendered in VR because I could have just as easily shot the man on a 2-D screen. The VR felt gratuitous. The visualizations were low resolution and unconvincing. The sound effects were laughable. It felt like I was trapped in a 3-D version of *Pong*. I wondered whether any patients had been consulted in the process of developing the program.

After many similar experiences with other ineffective programs, our research team decided in 2018 that it was time to establish formal guidelines for developing and validating VR treatments, just as there are standards for drug treatments. Led by Brandon Birckhead, a research scientist on our team at Cedars-Sinai, we convened an international group called the VR Clinical Outcomes Research Experts, or VR-CORE, and tapped the group's wisdom to develop best practices for assessing immersive therapeutics. The multidisciplinary group included experts in software design, clinical trials, epidemiology, and statistics. We also invited clinical experts in medicine, pediatrics, surgery, psychology, psychiatry, neuroscience, pain medicine, nursing, and rehabilitation.

Our goal was to offer guidance that would help developers avoid creating ineffective, poorly designed, and downright bad VR treatments. Hopefully, if we were successful, the result would be the opposite— more high-quality and effective treatments to fill the shelves of the VR pharmacy.

Before formalizing any guidance, we started by posing a simple question to our panel of experts: "When you think about the current state of clinical VR research, what comes to mind?" The feedback indicated there was room for improvement. One expert described therapeutic VR as the "Wild West" with a "lack of clear guidelines and standards." Another characterized the research as "heterogeneous" and often focused "more on the tech rather than the theories behind it." Overall, the committee expressed concerns that some of the research is overly descriptive, sometimes lacks enough participants to draw meaningful conclusions, and often fails to employ proper experimental designs. Although there are many outstanding research studies, such as the trials I've emphasized throughout this book, the committee believed that advancing the science of immersive therapeutics will require even more high-quality studies.

After a year of deliberation, we disseminated the group's recommendations in a 2019 peer-reviewed publication.[11] The result was a new framework describing three types of VR studies, called VR1, VR2, and VR3 trials. These are akin to the FDA Phase I–III trials that govern drug therapies. VR1 studies focus on developing VR content in partnership with patients, similar to the process we followed for So-HELP. VR2 trials are early tests of a treatment's feasibility, acceptability, and tolerability. VR3 studies are randomized, controlled trials that compare clinical outcomes between one group receiving the VR treatment and another receiving a control treatment.

The VR1 trial is especially vital because if it's not done right, then the subsequent trials are likely to fail for lack of involving patients early in the development cycle. The VR-CORE committee defined *three key principles* of VR1 trials.

First, VR designers should *promote empathy* in the development of a new treatment. That means carefully listening to and elucidating patients' needs, fears, habits, and expectations. The more time and effort developers commit in this early phase of development, the more likely they are to design a meaningful and effective VR treatment.

In the case of So-HELP, Coleman and her team conducted focus groups to understand health education needs, explore barriers to following a healthy diet, and learn how VR might lower blood pressure in the church community. The team learned that many people did not appreciate the importance of salt avoidance because high blood pressure—the major consequence of a high-salt diet—is a symptomless disease. Although catastrophic outcomes like stroke or heart attack might occur, many participants considered those to be theoretical outcomes; reducing salt was a big ask for managing an otherwise silent condition like hypertension.

When our VR team conferred with Coleman, we decided to create a virtual environment that acknowledged the difficulty of following a low-salt diet but still emphasized that dietary decisions can save lives. For example, here is the voice-over script for the scene where users enter their own chest cavity and confront their beating heart up close and personal:

> Wonderful, isn't it? Such an amazing organ. It can beat more than seventy times a minute for over a century. This heart is healthy at the moment. But, we're going to change that. I want you to see what happens to the heart when excessive sodium intake damages the walls of the arteries. Let's bring on the salt.

Then the arteries around the heart progressively lose color and become thinner. The heart begins to struggle and beats irregularly. The organ looks sickly. The heart sounds become weaker. The heart is failing. The narrator chimes in with some ideas for avoiding this fate:

> The heart is obviously vital to your health and there's a lot you can do to help it do its job. Physical activity if you're able, of course. Reducing sodium is an easy place to start as well. So maybe next time, pay attention to how many chips you've eaten, and maybe even sometimes, skip them altogether. I know, and I agree, that's a big ask. But look at this magnificent machine. Look how hard it works for you. Is skipping a handful of chips once in a while too much to do to keep it healthy? I think we both know the answer to that.

With these words, So-HELP empathizes with the difficulty of adhering to a low-salt diet but also confronts the misperception that hypertension is a symptomless disease with theoretical consequences. The program leverages the presence of VR to embody the negative effects of a high-salt diet, allowing users to experience their body in a new and viscerally arresting way. The silent killer of hypertension becomes visible and literally in your face. The lessons of So-HELP may not be pleasant, but they can be lifesaving. And what can be more empathic than designing a program that saves lives?

The second VR1 principle is to *promote team collaboration* when creating a new VR treatment. VR-CORE emphasizes that design teams should work together to generate as many ideas as they can, ranging from conservative and feasible to outright zany and ambitious. Just think about *TRIPP*. I can only imagine the design meeting when someone suggested that users fly around the metallic torso of a woman with glowing cheekbones and neon green hair, then view little floating orbs with photos of family members. And then everyone nodded knowingly, as if that was exactly what they were thinking, too.

By encouraging team collaboration and openness to ideas in the early stages of program development, VR-CORE wants design teams to think expansively and creatively rather than in a restrictive and conservative manner. Team members should be encouraged to generate ideas without being judged. Only then, after enumerating a full list of ideas, should the team cull out the most appropriate concepts for prototyping within technical and budgetary constraints.

The third VR1 principle is that treatments should be developed through *continuous user feedback* and iterative prototyping. This approach enables teams to rapidly test their ideas while incorporating real-time assessment from end users. Prototypes should be refined with continuous testing by patients. Failures should be viewed as an opportunity to learn and improve the prototype.

In contrast to a VR1 trial, which is focused on content development in a design environment, the VR2 trial evaluates what happens when the VR treatment is used by patients within the intended clinical setting. For example, a VR treatment focused on inpatient pain should be tested in a hospital environment. Another treatment targeting outpatient stroke rehabilitation should be evaluated in a physical therapy center or at a home setting. VR2 trials evaluate the acceptability, feasibility, and tolerability of the treatment in the natural setting where it is intended to be used.

In the context of a VR2 trial, *acceptability* refers to a patient's willingness to use the VR treatment. We saw in Chapter 6 that many patients express reservations about using VR, particularly while hospitalized or under duress. Patients may express skepticism, fear, or a sense of vulnerability, or they just might not want to be bothered by using the equipment. In a VR2 trial, investigators study whether patients are willing to try the VR treatment and collect information on why they did, or did not, find the treatment to be acceptable.

Distinct from acceptability, *feasibility* is the degree to which a VR treatment can be successfully integrated within the flow of usual care. Even the best designed VR treatments face implementation challenges when applied on the front lines of healthcare delivery. It is wise for developers to understand potential barriers, identify workarounds and solutions to these barriers, and only then consider testing their intervention in a VR3 trial. With So-HELP, for example, we learned quickly that the first version of the program was not ready for prime time. The participants found the instructions to be unclear, the navigation through the worlds to be confusing, and the equipment hard to use. I remember the day when we first unveiled VR to the parishioners. It was a mess. We ran around from table to table troubleshooting the software, rebooting the computers, and answering questions from nearly every participant about how to operate the hardware and software. We thought the program had been sufficiently beta tested in the lab, but it turned out to be far from ready. It took several rounds of iterative prototyping before we could feel confident the program would serve its intended purpose.

Next comes *tolerability*. The VR2 trial offers an early opportunity to evaluate whether the treatment causes any side effects, such as cybersickness, DP/DR symptoms, or other unanticipated consequences. Researchers should also test for any discomfort or inconvenience from the VR equipment itself, such as ill-fitting headsets, facial or nasal pain, or an inability to fully explore 3-D environments due to limited mobility.

Finally comes the VR3 trial. This definitive clinical test is a prospective, large, scientifically rigorous randomized trial that evaluates clinical outcomes and safety. When performed correctly, a VR3 trial should standardize the intervention, precisely specify the intended patient population, select an appropriate control condition, allocate subjects between conditions using a random number generator, measure clinically relevant outcomes over a sufficient period of time, apply appropriate statistical analyses, and, importantly, be registered in a publicly accessible online study databank.

"We don't want people selling snake oil out there," Brandon Birckhead tells me. Brandon is the lead author of the VR-CORE guidelines, who also says, "For a doctor, payer, or regulator like the FDA to get behind a VR treatment, they need to know the program is evidence-based, rigorously developed, and fit-for-purpose." If more developers use the VR-CORE framework to design their VR treatments, then higher quality, more effective, and safer offerings will appear in the VR pharmacy.

Melissa Wong, the obstetrician using VR during childbirth, agrees. "Sometimes I wonder if anyone is asking patients for their opinion on this stuff," she lamented to me in an interview. "I mean, the first randomized trial of VR for laboring women used a manatee bobbing around in the water as the distraction experience. Here you've got women in their most manatee-like state, all swollen up and trying to deliver a baby, and you show them a huge manatee? Seriously? What are they supposed to do, summon their inner manatee while giving birth? I can only imagine what the focus groups would say about that."

Wong worked with software developer AppliedVR to test a more tailored program for childbirth based on the experiences of Erin Martucci, the first woman to give birth aided by VR, whom we met back in Chapter 3. The original program that Erin used promoted slow, rhythmic breathing, similar to Lamaze breathing, to help her engage during the birth of her child. Wong now uses a similar version of the program, but it has been enhanced with a voice-over that is customized for childbirth. "Rather than playing some random music or pumping in the sounds of a manatee or whatever," Wong explains, "the software talks to the woman as she labors and offers relevant motivations." The program includes a menu of seven experiences that users can select while progressing through labor. In one module, called "Reassuring," the audio guide offers tailored advice:

> Remember, you are healthy and have all you need to go through labor. You are strong and flexible. You are able to adapt and adjust. You know how to do this. Your baby knows how to do this. Labor works. Your body works. Find harmony in your mind and in your heart. You are in good hands. You are in control of your labor. You can adjust its pace. Reassure your baby it is okay to come down, that you are ready to meet.

Whether it's minding the progress of labor, meditating with family members, or learning healthy eating from a pastor, precision immersion puts the patient in the center. When VR is personalized, the results can be profound, not only while the patient is in the headset but also well after they remove the goggles.

Juanita Cannon, a parishioner at Holman Church who used VR to control her blood pressure, is a case in point. When a crew from the CBS

Evening News came through the church to cover the So-HELP study, they asked Cannon to look into the headset and describe what she saw.

"Oh Lord," she exclaimed, looking at a virtual plate of lasagna. "Two thousand milligrams of salt, my god!"[12] Cannon was standing in the virtual kitchen surrounded by meals that looked familiar. They were familiar, of course, because Cannon and her fellow parishioners had built that kitchen from the ground up together with Coleman, Sauls, and our VR team.

"When you actually see what's going on, that opens your eyes," she said.

Prior to using VR, Cannon would salt all her food liberally. After, she began to lightly season her food with a pinch. She didn't need to be in VR to cook differently. The personalized environment brought the cooking lessons to life and, "So-HELP me God," says Sauls, might even promote a longer and healthier life.

As the VR pharmacy grows and the role of immersive therapy expands across healthcare, it will become routine for virtualists to help manage a panoply of diseases. Precision immersion will allow doctors to pick the right program for the right patient at the right time. There will be less emphasis on generic, impersonalized treatment protocols, and more focus on using evidence-based, FDA-cleared treatments borne from rigorous scientific inquiry. If we are careful to acknowledge and respect the patient's voice in creating and prescribing new treatments, VR can strengthen the humanity in healing.

In Part I: Our Bodies, Our Selves, we learned about the science of immersive therapeutics. In Part II: Virtual Medicine, we learned about the practice. Now it's time to explore the future. In Part III: Brave New World we will study how the vision of humanistic VR can make doctors more empathic with their patients, and make patients more empathic with themselves.

Brave New World

VR connects humans to other humans in a profound way that I've never seen before in any other form of media. And it can change people's perception of each other. And that's how I think virtual reality has the potential to actually change the world.

—Chris Milk, immersive artist and VR innovator

CHAPTER TEN

The Empathy Machine

I AM STANDING IN A MODEST APARTMENT WITH WHITE WALLS, A RED carpet, and a wooden table. There is a mirror on the wall by the front entrance. A man walks through the door and enters the room. He is wearing a brown sweater, dark jeans, and a look of disgust. As I face him, I notice my reflection staring back from the mirror behind the man's looming profile. But the person in the mirror is not me; it is a woman. I look down at my body and see a female figure. I am not accustomed to these shapes. I'm not used to someone lowering his gaze to meet my eyes. I am no longer me. I have embodied a young woman, and now I am on the receiving end of a long, hard stare from a very tall and unhappy man.

"What are you doing?" he asks.

"Uh, nothing," I reply.

"Shut up!"

I avert my eyes for a minute and stare at my reflection in the mirror. He notices.

"Look at me!" he commands.

There is a long pause. The man runs his eyes up and down my body.

"Have you realized how ugly you look? Where are you going dressed like that? I think you could dress a little bit better. No? You look twenty years older in those clothes."

I don't reply. I can still see myself in the mirror, just standing there with his foreboding figure reflected from behind. He hurls more insults at me, raising his voice as he slowly walks closer. I begin to feel cornered, even helpless. There is a telephone on the table beside him. He picks it up.

"You like talking on the phone, don't you? You know what I'm going to say to you? This is going to end. Do you see the phone? Do you see it? This phone is going to hell!"

He smashes the phone against the wall in a violent fit. Now he comes even closer. He's right on top of me and invading my personal space. He is taller than me by a good half a foot. He trains his eyes on mine, furrows his brow, and grits his teeth.

"Because all this is my fault. . . . All this is my fault. Because I have been very nice to you . . . very patient. And why? Because I love you. I love you." He raises his hand, as if he's about to strike me. And then . . .

I take off my VR headset and, once again, find myself back in Mel Slater's lab in Barcelona where I am safe and sound. But my mind is reverberating from what just happened. I was just a victim of domestic violence. I cannot pretend to know the pain of victimhood, but somehow, this vivid scenario feels all too real.

The domestic violence simulator not only provides a glimpse of what it's like to be a victim, but it also can subject perpetrators to their own abuse. The Catalan Department of Justice now encourages domestic violence offenders to experience the simulator from the perspective of a victim as part of their state-mandated rehabilitation program. The results have been remarkable.

In a 2018 study titled "Offenders Become the Victim in Virtual Reality: Impact of Changing Perspective in Domestic Violence," led by Mavi Sanchez-Vives, researchers subjected twenty male perpetrators to the VR simulation and compared their responses to a control group of nonviolent men.[1] Before entering VR, participants in both groups completed a psychological test to see how well they could read the emotional expression of women's faces that flashed by as images on a screen. Compared to the control group, the offenders were less able to detect a fearful demeanor and were more likely to confuse fear with happiness. The violent men were handicapped at reading emotions, which helps explain, in part, why they committed their crimes in the first place.[2] However, after embodying a female victim and being intimidated and abused by the virtual bully, the perpetrators improved their ability to read emotions during post-VR testing. In contrast, the nonviolent men were accurate both before and after the simulation. Sanchez-Vives concluded that "changing the perspective of an aggressive population by means of virtual embodiment in the victim impacts emotional recognition." VR created space for these violent men to act with greater empathy. Although the study did not track long-term outcomes, low rates of recidivism have been found among parolees who completed the virtual rehabilitation program in a preliminary study, suggesting durable benefits well after removing the headsets.[3]

The Catalonian study reveals another unique capability of VR: It enables perspective-taking. And perspective-taking is the key to empathizing. We empathize with people when we see the world through their eyes and acknowledge their experiences. Sharing the first-person perspective of another person in distress cultivates compassion. That's how I felt after experiencing the domestic violence simulator. Thankfully, I have never been beaten or abused. I have never been told to dress differently because I look ugly, have never been knowingly regarded as an inanimate object, and have never had a phone thrown at me. But the VR simulator caused me to mentally rehearse those experiences. Now, when I hear a story like Gloria's, which we considered in Chapter 8, or when I learn that one of my patients has been abused, I think back to that time in Slater's lab. I have a mental anchor that causes me to stop and regard what it means to be a victim of abuse. It causes me to think differently because I've now seen a perpetrator come at me with my own eyes. I've heard an abuser yell at me with my own ears. I cannot know the pain of being a victim, but I have at least embodied the role in a simulation.

Other VR researchers around the world are leveraging the power of perspective-taking. For example, studies reveal that when light-skinned people experience living in a dark-skinned body, it reduces implicit bias against racial and ethnic minorities.[4] Other research shows that virtual embodiment can boost empathy for people who are homeless, for maltreated children, for Syrian refugees, and for the elderly.[5] This effect of VR is so extensible that it can even cause embodiment of nonhuman forms. In one study led by Jeremy Bailenson at Stanford University, scientists used VR to make people feel like a cow being prodded, poked, and then shipped to the slaughterhouse.[6] In another study by the same team, people watched the exhaust from their vehicle percolate into the ocean, increase carbon dioxide levels in the water, and destroy the coral reef. The study revealed how experiencing life in the ocean can elevate awareness about climate change.[7]

If VR can shift perspective so radically that it causes people to empathize with cows and coral, then maybe it could also instill more humanity into healing. As a doctor, I always try to empathize with my patients. But that's not always easy because it is difficult to know what my patients are truly experiencing. I do not know what it's like to be blind or to have advanced dementia or to have schizophrenia. I have not felt the paralysis of stroke. I have not been wheeled into an operating room for emergency surgery. I take care of many people with IBS, but I don't *really* know what it feels like to have abdominal pain, stomach cramps, and diarrhea every day. I can only imagine what that's like. This is where VR can make a difference. I have felt differently about domestic violence ever since visiting Slater's lab in Barcelona. Perhaps I can feel differently about other conditions, too, with the help of other virtual environments.

Inspired by the work of empathy scientists like Bailenson, Sanchez-Vives, and Slater, medical VR researchers and software companies are now exploring how to promote empathy and strengthen the doctor-patient bond through VR. In one effort, doctors embody a patient with Parkinson's disease and experience three stages of the patient's life: living at home, where it becomes difficult for family members to care for the patient; meeting with a neurologist who delivers the diagnosis of Parkinson's; and transitioning to an assisted living community with other patients suffering from dementia.[8] The simulation was created by Carrie Shaw, CEO of Embodied Labs, who became a caregiver at a young age following her mother's diagnosis of early-onset dementia. She witnessed communication breakdowns and noticed that doctors often struggled to understand what her mother was seeing and feeling. Shaw created Embodied Labs as a way to offer doctors a new set of tools to engage with their patients. Her company is leveraging extensive research that shows VR improves knowledge retention, satisfaction, and engagement among doctors and medical students. "Our labs take learners from a passive to an active role where we literally put them into the shoes of the person with the disease," explains Shaw. "This holistic approach creates enhanced understanding, empathy and ultimately better quality of care."[9]

VR has been used to teach doctors what it's like to experience the progressive blindness of macular degeneration and glaucoma, to experience an acute migraine headache, to live in a hospice receiving palliative care for advanced cancer, to experience hallucinations, and to enter an MRI scanner while undergoing a critical imaging study. [10]

In one simulation developed at University College London, doctors sit face-to-face with a patient who is demanding antibiotics for a cold, but who the doctor doesn't think needs the remedy—a common scenario that taxes both patient and provider.[11] In the virtual world, doctors can practice communicating empathically with patients while emphasizing the risks of inappropriately prescribing needless antibiotics.

In another simulation created by researchers at the Hospital for Sick Children in Toronto, doctors feel what it's like to be placed on a gurney, rolled into an operating room, and administered anesthesia so that they can gain greater insight about the importance of empathic communication during a time of great anxiety.[12] A randomized controlled trial conducted at the medical college at Thomas Jefferson University in Philadelphia revealed that patients who use preoperative VR are more satisfied with their care and less stressed compared to patients who do not prepare in VR.[13]

In Chapter 6 we learned how George Engel's biopsychosocial model has changed the practice of medicine from a "doctor knows best" mentality based in biomedical thinking, to a model of shared decision-making between patients and their doctors. Here, we see how VR can enable Engel's vision by allowing doctors to walk a mile in their patients' shoes, better understand their life experiences, and leverage those insights to make shared decisions.

Medical schools are taking note. "It's impossible for a twenty-four-year-old medical student to understand what it's like to be someone sixty years older than themselves," says Carrie Shaw, whose company is now working to integrate its virtual empathy labs into medical school curricula.[14] At the University of New England College of Osteopathic Medicine, Shaw's VR labs were designated as required viewing for all the students. Elizabeth Dyer is an associate dean at the school who oversees the program and published the initial findings.[15] "Assessment results indicate that students demonstrate increased understanding of and empathy with older adults who have age-related conditions such as macular degeneration and hearing loss," she concluded. "Research indicates that empathy leads to better patient care and outcomes and that educational interventions work, so it is worthwhile to address this subject area in the curriculum."

In contrast to many other health technologies, which can distance doctors from their patients and undermine the human touch, immersion motivates doctors to confront the biopsychosocial illness of their patients and prompts discussions that might not otherwise happen in the absence of vivid perspective-taking. Young doctors-in-training can practice interviewing virtual patients in low-risk environments, learn how to empathize meaningfully and reproducibly, and cultivate enhanced emotional and social awareness about their patients' life experiences.

But the empathy boost is not just limited to patients and their providers. Research also shows that VR enables patients to empathize with another key stakeholder: themselves.

When Danielle Collins felt the worst headache of her life while in a Pilates class, she knew something was wrong. "It was like an ice pick driving through my skull," she would later recall. The pain didn't subside, so she went to her local emergency department at the George Washington

University Hospital in Washington, DC, where a CT scan revealed a bleed in her head the size of a softball. For an otherwise healthy and athletic twenty-seven-year-old, this was shocking and bewildering news.

The next hour presented a whirlwind of activity. Nurses started IVs, administered medicines, and checked her vital signs repeatedly. Doctors came in and out of her room. It became clear that Danielle was going to need brain surgery to stop the bleeding and save her life. She was terrified, confused, and struggling to piece everything together. "I didn't know what was happening," she later told me. "I didn't understand what was going on inside my head."

Then, in the midst of Danielle's personal chaos, Dr. Walter Jean, a professor of neurosurgery at George Washington, entered with a VR headset. "Do you want to fly," he asked? He handed the headset to Danielle, who put it on, opened her eyes, and came face-to-face with the fantastical vista of some alien planet: her brain. She flew straight through her skull, penetrated her own meninges, and arrived at a crimson red artery bleeding deep within her cerebral cortex.

"You have an arteriovenous malformation," Jean explained. "We're right on the surface of it now, so we have to eliminate all of that," he said, referring to the knotted tangle of blood vessels tucked away in her temporal lobe. Danielle hovered over the lesion, zooming in, and out, watching the blood enter and exit the area. She could see exactly where it was as Jean described the problem and discussed his plan to operate.

Jean was using a system called *Surgical Theater* that reconstructs CT scan images into virtual reality. Armed with a VR headset, Danielle could explore her own brain through a first-person view. "It gave me a completely new perspective on myself," Danielle told me when we met three years after that fateful day. "The result was amazing, because it created this experience where nothing was unknown anymore. It cut through the uncertainty. I could see what the problem was and know it could be fixed."

The surgery was successful. Dr. Jean removed the lesion and Danielle fully recovered. Now she's had time to reflect on what happened. "Ever since flying through my brain, I've never seen myself the same way. The VR made me more grateful for each and every moment that we have."

VR allowed Danielle to shift perspective, not about someone else's plight, but about her own plight. She saw herself differently, quite literally, and that radical frameshift transitioned Danielle from battling an existential crisis to calmly accepting that her mind and body were in good hands. Danielle's story shows how VR can offer us headspace not only to think differently about others, but to think differently about ourselves. Now, inspired by the unique capability of VR, scientists are finding other creative ways to use it as a self-empathy machine.

At UCLA, for example, researchers turned to VR to help patients with HIV think differently about their disease in an effort to boost medication adherence. Doctors had noticed that many HIV patients were struggling to stay on their lifesaving drugs because, in some cases, they did not understand how the medicines worked. In a remarkable 2019 study led by professor Omer Liran, patients with HIV watched a VR experience that allowed them to fly into their body and learn about their illness.[16] Using a first-person perspective, the patients entered their virtual arteries and encountered bacteria spreading green poisonous particles into the blood. Next, a white blood cell floated by and engulfed the bacteria, clearing the pathogens from the bloodstream. But before long, an HIV virus came through, entered the white blood cell, and caused it to explode—a scene made even more dramatic with ominous music. The bacteria escaped and the arteries turned green, indicating progressive illness. Then the scene reset, hopeful music replaced the dark score, and a narrator encouraged the patient to press a button "to release a dose of lifesaving medicine." With the button engaged, brilliant gold particles entered the artery and formed a shield around the white blood cell that repulsed a swarm of HIV. The narrator explained that the medicine worked and the body had healed, but the patient had to stay on the medicine in order to maintain the protective shield.

The VR program did more than improve patients' knowledge about HIV and its treatment: patients took more of their lifesaving medicine, which led to objectively lower viral levels and a measurably strengthened immune system. Liran concluded that "compared with other traditional media platforms such as videos, VR is more immersive and thus has a greater positive emotional impact, which can improve engagement and learning." Once again, it was the emotional impact of VR that mattered. Handing out a trifold brochure or having patients watch a 2-D video might not have made as much of a difference. Instead, VR allowed patients to see themselves differently, understand themselves differently, and gain healthy new perspectives that endured long after removing the headset.

What's happening in these moments? Is VR empathy an ineffable feeling, or is it something we can directly observe? If we had a way of measuring the biomarkers of VR empathy, then maybe developers could custom-build software that fosters compassion for the self and others.

An evolving field of science called empathic neurofeedback seeks to measure and leverage the physiologic signals of human compassion.[17] In a typical experiment, researchers expose subjects to beautiful music or an emotional cinematic experience and monitor their brain with an electroencephalogram (EEG). Using that approach, scientists discovered that empathic feelings tend to correlate with the appearance of alpha waves spread around the front of the brain in an asymmetric pattern.[18] (You might recall we discussed flow-inducing alpha waves back in Chapter 2). Neurofeedback researchers are now using programs to detect these empathy signals and feed the results into a VR headset to deliver synchronized virtual environments, similar to Adam Gazzaley's sensory immersion vessel described in Chapter 5. By using a brain-computer interface system like Gazzaley's, neurofeedback scientists hope to teach people new ways of recognizing and augmenting their inner capacity to empathize.[19]

But there's one very simple, universal, and easily observable sign of empathy that can be measured without fancy neuroimaging equipment: goose bumps. When goose bumps occur from an emotional experience, rather than from just feeling cold, they are called psychogenic shivering—a technical term for getting the chills. Some people have more psychogenic shivering ability than others, but you've almost certainly felt it at some point in your life. The chills usually start between the shoulder blades at the top of your back and then extend down your arms. They may accompany a perception of awe, a sense of altruism, and a feeling of openness or profound meaning around the triggering event. People often experience goose bumps during transformative experiences, such as attending a wedding, participating in a religious or spiritual event, or hearing awe-inspiring music. Goose bumps may even indicate an aha moment when a worldview changes, not just in positive environments but also in negative circumstances.[20]

Cognitive scientists are now using VR to trigger and measure goose bumps as an outward sign of empathy. In a creative study titled "Are You Awed Yet? How Virtual Reality Gives Us Awe and Goose Bumps," Denise Quesnel and Bernhard Riecke from Simon Fraser University used a "goosecam" to record a patch of forearm skin as subjects orbited Earth in virtual reality.[21] Their goal was to recreate the awe and humility frequently described by astronauts when confronted with the vastness of our planet, and then to test whether that transcendent experience could provoke psychogenic shivers.[22]

It turns out that VR could deliver the willies. When Quesnel and Riecke fired up their VR space capsule, they recorded goose bumps in 44 percent of participants within minutes of starting the journey (67 percent of women and 30 percent of men got the chills). When participants experienced goose bumps, they were also more likely to report subjective experiences of awe, wonder, curiosity, and humility, indicating that the physical response correlated with the mental response. Many people experienced a shift in perception during their simulated space flight. Some described changes to their moral attitude. Others mentioned changes in how they view the environment, or how they perceive their own problems in comparison to the vastness of humanity. Still others felt a new sense of empathy for people in the world experiencing a challenging way of life. "Since awe is thought to generate a shift in self-concept in how a person sees themselves in the world," wrote Quesnel and Riecke, "exploring shifts in self-concept generated through a virtual environment may provide helpful frameworks."

Other scientists are finding new ways to foster empathy by leveraging the chill-inducing properties of VR. In one notable example, a multidisciplinary team from Europe and the United States created a "wearable chill-actuator" that stirs up shivers at just the right moment during a VR experience.[23] The goose bump machine sends concentrated vibrations and thermoelectric cooling waves along the upper back on demand, causing users to literally feel the chills. This way, scientists can dial up goose bumps at a predefined moment to cultivate a sense of empathy for those who might not ordinarily feel the shivers.

"What's wrong in healthcare today," says Eric Topol, noted physician and author, "is that it's missing care."[24] In the current era of big data analytics, artificial intelligence, and algorithmic diagnostics, many doctors routinely complain that technology disrupts the physician-patient relationship and undermines the art of empathic medicine. Research indicates that doctors now spend more time conducting desktop medicine—that is, staring at a computer screen—than practicing bedside medicine, where they look patients in the eyes.[25]

But the examples noted in this chapter reveal how VR flips desktop medicine on its head. In contrast to technologies that require doctors to stare at screens in lieu of facing their patients, VR reminds doctors to focus on their patients and consider their inner lives. It prompts doctors to consider the subjective nature of illness and enables patient-centered dialogue. As Engel's biopsychosocial model continues to penetrate medicine, VR takes on greater significance as an empathy machine that connects doctors and patients in more meaningful and lasting ways.

The longer I work in immersive therapeutics, the more strongly I believe that it's not a computer science or an engineering science, but a social and behavioral science. It is not about the latest gadgets and gizmos, but about leveraging technology to foster altruism, awe, and compassion. When used with the right people, in the right way, and at the right time, VR strengthens the humanity in healing like no other technology.

CHAPTER ELEVEN

Through the Looking Glass

T'S 8:00 A.M. ON MONDAY AND MY INBOX IS FILLING UP WITH CON-
sults. There's a list of patients in the hospital waiting to be seen by our
team of virtualists. We're ready to get the day started.

The first patient is Candice, a thirty-one-year-old woman with fibromyalgia and severe lower back pain. Fibromyalgia can be a devastating
disease. It causes pain throughout the body and leaves patients feeling fatigued, overwhelmed, and often depressed. Candice has a severe case that
has required several hospitalizations and opioids. But the treatment isn't
working. Now she's back in the hospital and looking for help.

Candice was just admitted yesterday. Within minutes of entering
the hospital, a computer algorithm had already spotted some concerning
trends. The system noticed multiple readmissions and rising pain scores
despite an escalating dose of opioids. It also detected a new prescription
for laxatives, which indicates the opioids may be slowing her digestion.
These findings triggered the computer to hot-spot Candice for closer

assessment. Wasting no time, the system immediately notified her doctor that Candice is at high risk for opioid use disorder and may benefit from alternative treatments, including VR therapy. The doctor agreed, clicked a button on the screen to consult the virtualists, and sent over a digital request. And now we're on the case.

We meet Candice in her room. She is lying in bed and clearly distressed. There is an IV in her arm delivering high-dose narcotics, but she is still grimacing in pain. We discuss the role of VR for pain control and review how it might offer benefits as a nondrug therapy. We can't promise that VR will replace her pain meds, but we discuss how it might help lower the dose. Candice is up for anything. She's willing to give it a try.

We hand her a tablet computer with a program designed to optimize VR treatment based on her unique preferences. There are twelve different images on the screen ranging from dolphins swimming in the ocean to the Redwood Forest to a Hawaiian beach to the Grand Canyon. "Look closely at all the pictures," the computer instructs, "and then select one that makes you feel most peaceful inside."

After some thought, Candice taps on an image of a forest and up come several more options. Now she can add a river to the scene, or a meadow, or maybe a lake. She can sprinkle in grazing deer, turn the clock to dawn or dusk, add clouds and birds to the sky, or even make it rain. She selects her ideal scene after a few minutes of tinkering. The tablet electronically sends her preferences to the hospital computer system, which relays the information to a cabinet full of VR headsets in the nursing station down the hall. The cabinet is much more than a storage unit: it charges, sanitizes, and personalizes VR headsets for each patient on the ward. The headset assigned to Candice receives her preference profile along with a library of pain management programs.

But we also want to address the opioid side effects. The meds are paralyzing her bowels and causing severe constipation that requires high-dose laxatives. To help manage the problem, we start by placing a small biosensor on her abdomen right near the belly button. The sensor sticks onto the skin and has a microphone that listens to the rumbling of her bowels; it uses the acoustic signals to calculate a vital sign called the intestinal rate, which is the number of intestinal contractions per minute.

As digestion picks up, so does the intestinal rate. But as digestion slows down—or even becomes paralyzed from the opioids—the intestinal rate slows in lockstep and the belly becomes quiet.

Using closed-loop biofeedback between the sensor and VR headset, we can now measure Candice's bowel sounds and instantly transmit the results back into her virtual environment. As the opioids kick in and her digestion halts, the river flowing through her virtual forest slows down, eventually becoming a stagnant swamp once the bowels are paralyzed. When the opioids wear off and her digestion speeds up, so does the river. Now Candice can see exactly what's happening in her belly and use the feedback to make better decisions about whether, when, and how much to use the meds. We explain to Candice that we will electronically track her progress and return tomorrow to see if it's helping her pain or reducing the opioid dose.

We need to keep moving, so we leave the medical ward and head over to the neurology unit to visit our next patient, Sophia, who is a twenty-five-year-old woman with a brain tumor. Thankfully, the tumor is benign and does not pose a mortal risk. But it is located in an area that has left Sophia almost completely blind. She can only see through a small circle of remaining vision in her right eye, and what little she can make out is blurry. Surgeons are concerned about removing the tumor because it is so deep in her brain. In the meantime, they are seeking nonsurgical ways to bolster her vision. They call in our team for help.

We decide to try a low vision enhancement system, or LVES, which is a form of VR therapy that magnifies images to compensate for diminished sight. The LVES employs a headset with a high-resolution video camera mounted in front of the goggles that can expand selected regions of its forward-facing view. Because Sophia still has a small patch of remaining vision, we program the LVES to telescope in on that precise area of viable sight. A computer program clarifies blurred edges, enhances contrast between objects, and expands her tiny viewing portal tenfold to fill the entire stereoscopic image in the VR headset.

With all the adjustments complete, we present Sophia with a writing sample to see if she can make out the words. She hasn't been able to read anything for the past two months. At first she struggles to see the text. The LVES hasn't quite trained its magnification onto the right spot. Now she uses a hand controller to precisely dial in the final adjustments. She taps the magnification window slightly left, jogs it slightly up, and pauses for a moment as our team anxiously awaits her report.

"Can you see it?" asks her neurologist.

"Yeah . . ." she replies. "Yeah, I can see it."

"What do you see?"

"Oh my god, it's amazing!" Sophia gathers herself and reads the entire writing sample. She looks around the room and begins to describe what she sees. The LVES is working. It has not removed her tumor, nor has it cured her disease. But like Alice in *Through the Looking-Glass*, Sophia stares into a fantastical world beyond the lens. For now, at least, her vision is restored.

Down the hall there is another patient in the neurology ward awaiting our visit. Marcus is a sixty-two-year-old man with high blood pressure and diabetes who recently suffered a stroke that paralyzed the right side of his body. His physical rehabilitation has been slow and doctors are looking to accelerate progress.

After reviewing his case, we determine that Marcus is an ideal candidate for VR stroke therapy. We begin by placing motion sensors on his hands and affixing VR goggles on his head through which he views a first-person avatar of his body. Marcus now sees and feels his arms resting on a table placed across his hospital bed. There is a virtual blue ball on the corner of the table. We ask Marcus to grab it with his right hand, but the paralysis blocks his will to move.

"This time try moving your left hand instead," instructs Dr. Brandon Birckhead, the virtualist assigned to Marcus's case. "See if you can reach the ball with your healthy arm."

"Okay," Marcus replies. As expected, he moves his left hand effortlessly. But unexpectedly, Marcus's left hand doesn't move in VR; it's his *right* hand that reaches for the ball.

"Whoa!"

"What do you see?" asks Birckhead.

"I just moved my right hand! I grabbed the ball!"

The VR system reversed his hands in the virtual world. Now, by moving his healthy left arm, Marcus controls his paralyzed right arm across the virtual table. The visual feedback convinces Marcus's brain that his right hand is healthy and strong.

As Marcus continues to experiment with his virtual limb reversal, we notice something important is happening back in real reality. When Marcus moves his left hand, his paralyzed right hand begins to twitch ever so slightly. His brain is sending signals to the paralyzed limb. It's an early flicker of hope that brain and body can reconnect. This is a great prognostic sign. Dr. Birckhead prescribes a VR treatment program that Marcus and his team will follow for the next several weeks. We plan to check back to monitor his progress.

We're running behind schedule, so it's time to head over to our outpatient clinic where more consults await. We take the elevator downstairs, exit the hospital, and cross the street to the virtualist clinic where the lobby is full with patients scheduled for immersive therapeutics.

Our first outpatient, Ramone, is a sixty-eight-year-old man who suffered a heart attack two months ago that was successfully treated by opening a blocked coronary artery. Now he's taking a bevy of medicines to keep the blood flowing and lower his chances of another event. But medicines alone won't be enough to ensure that Ramone stays healthy. He also needs to exercise regularly while keeping within the constraints of his healing heart. That's why his doctors enrolled Ramone in our VR cardiac rehab program. Today is his second week coming to the virtual gym.

We place a wireless heart monitor on his chest and an oxygenation probe over his index finger. He dons a VR headset and grabs hold of a controller in each hand. Ramone opens his eyes and the white-walled clinic is now replaced by a dark chamber with neon-highlighted cubes emerging at full speed from a distant horizon. He is holding a light saber in each of his hands, one blue, one red. As the cubes barrel toward him, Ramone sizes up their trajectory and prepares to slice each cube in half using the sabers. Blue cubes must be cut by the blue saber, and red cubes by the red saber. Each cube has an arrow indicating the direction of the slice, causing Ramone to lunge around from side to side, constantly trying to keep up with the incoming barrage of objects as high-energy club music plays in his ears. Before long, his heart is racing and he's breathing quickly.

A computer closely monitors Ramone's progress and ensures that he stays within the physiologic bounds set by his cardiologist. The computer slows the pace whenever his vital signs stray above the prescribed range, allowing Ramone to fall back into a safe rhythm for his heart. If his activity drops below the range, then the computer picks up the pace, challenging him to push harder and faster, but always within the desired parameters. He takes a breather after thirty minutes and reviews his score. The data reveal that Ramone performed 12 percent better than his last workout in the VR gym. He is making verifiable progress while also staying safe. Ramone will come back on Wednesday for his next round of virtual Jedi training.

Next up is Sarah, a thirty-five-year-old woman with depression and anxiety who is using VR to supplement antidepressants prescribed by her psychiatrist. Today, she is reporting for a virtual counseling session in our clinic. Sarah sits down on a couch, puts on a headset, and finds herself on a beach sitting across from Mother Teresa.

"This week has been a little better," Sarah says.

"I'm glad to hear that," Mother Teresa replies.

"But I'm still feeling down at night. That's when I realize how lonely I feel sitting in my apartment."

"That must be difficult."

"Yeah, it's hard."

Sarah and Mother Teresa continue to talk back and forth. Throughout the dialogue, sensors are measuring Sarah's heart rate variability, eye motion, respirations, and galvanic skin resistance, offering clues about her emotional state. Mother Teresa is monitoring the feedback and using the results to guide the conversation.

But Mother Teresa is not a human; she's a *virtual human* guided by artificial intelligence. Sarah chose Mother Teresa to be her therapeutic avatar, but a computer is driving the conversation and fine-tuning every aspect of the talk therapy, from the question stems to the tone of voice to the length of pauses between statements. Our team is standing by to offer our own voice, as needed, but Mother Teresa takes the lead. When Sarah goes home, she'll take Mother Teresa with her and continue VR therapy outside of the clinic. We'll check back next week to see how she's doing.

Our last patient of the day is in the virtual rehab unit receiving treatment for a severe spinal cord injury. Ever since falling from a ladder fourteen months ago, Omar, a forty-two-year-old construction worker, has been paralyzed from the waist down. But lately, with the help of VR and a robotic exoskeleton, he is showing signs of recovery. Today we're checking up on his progress.

When we meet Omar he is standing upright with the help of a suspension system that has been lowered from the ceiling. There are arm rails on either side that he's using to help support his body. He is wearing a sixteen-channel EEG on his head that is measuring brain waves across both cerebral hemispheres. And on his face is a VR headset that is beaming him a first-person view of his digitized body.

"Okay, now imagine lifting your right leg," instructs his physical therapist.

Omar wills his leg to move. The EEG senses the brain waves and triggers movement of his right leg in the virtual environment.

"Great, now lift your left leg."

Once again, the EEG detects Omar's will to move, this time lifting his digitized left leg. From Omar's perspective, he can see his legs moving smoothly and naturally in synchrony with the commands from his brain. He feels like he's walking, although it's all within a virtual world.

Next, his physical therapy team helps Omar into an elaborate robotic exoskeleton that looks like something from an Iron Man movie. Omar's legs are surrounded by mechanical actuators that are custom-fitted around his joints and designed to bend his legs into a natural gait. The device includes pressure pads that apply force to strategic locations along his limbs, including the surface of his feet, knees, and hips, to simulate the tactile feedback of walking that able-bodied people take for granted.

"Where do you want to walk today?" asks the therapist.

"Pan Pacific Park," he replies. "I used to play soccer there as a kid."

The technicians pull up a view of the park from Google Earth and display 360-degree images in Omar's head-mounted display. Now he's on the soccer field at his childhood park. He looks down and sees his healthy body. A soccer ball rolls up to his feet. Omar imagines kicking the ball with his right foot, triggering brain waves that instruct the exoskeleton to move his right leg toward the virtual ball. He imagines chasing after the ball, and that's exactly what he does in both virtual reality, where he sees himself running, and in real reality, where the exoskeleton articulates his body across the floor.

It's going to take time, but we hope that Omar will eventually regain some ability to walk. He's been in the VR rehab program for several months and has a long road ahead. In the meantime, he is showing signs of steady recovery, not only in the virtual world, but also in the real, physical world. Time will tell if both worlds converge into one reality.

It's been a long day and we're ready to head home. Tomorrow starts anew and, no doubt, we'll have more consults waiting when we return in the morning.

You might have guessed by now that this vision of virtual medicine is, for the moment, hypothetical. But it is all possible. Science is not a barrier to implementing this vision of virtual medicine. The barriers are more mundane, like a lack of staffing, infrastructure, and funding. What we need now is a dose of vision and a can of elbow grease.

Consider Candice. Every bit of her story is possible right now. For starters, all modern hospitals now use an electronic health record to monitor their patients. This ubiquitous resource enables programmers to run algorithms that spot patients who need special care. For example, my team developed a program that alerts doctors about patients at risk for opioid dependency; to help reduce adverse outcomes it offers recommendations, like referring patients to opioid abatement programs or generating an opioid use agreement for doctors to review with their patients.[1] Programming this type of clinical decision support is now trivial and can be used to identify patients like Candice who might benefit from VR. This approach is similar to the idea noted in Chapter 9 of using computerized regression analysis to detect patients eligible for VR treatment. Candice was also able to personalize her treatment with a tablet computer using a form of conjoint analysis—the preference assessment technique we also covered in Chapter 9.

What about the abdominal biosensor? That's also not science fiction. Years ago I co-invented a wearable sensor called AbStats that was cleared by the FDA to monitor bowel sounds.[2] The sensor listens to rumbling in the belly and converts the noise into a signal that doctors use to monitor gut activity. Connecting AbStats to a VR headset is straightforward and conceptually no different than Adam Gazzaley's sensory immersion vessel or Les Posen's airplane phobia setup described in Chapter 5; all are examples of closed-loop biofeedback that couple sensors to a virtual environment. Whether it's heart rate, respirations, blood pressure, or bowel sounds, doctors can employ all forms of biodata to customize responsive virtual worlds. I believe the future of immersive therapeutics will feature many more examples of closed-loop biofeedback.

What about Sophia's story? Can VR actually restore sight? Several companies are now developing and selling low-vision enhancement systems for people like Sophia.[3] In fact, Sophia's story is based on a real patient, named Maisy, who uses an LVES built by the British company GiveVision. Maisy has a brain tumor that rendered her legally blind for six years prior to discovering the GiveVision goggles. She first used the device onstage at the 2019 Hay Festival in England while being recorded by national media. Spencer Kelly, the stage moderator, handed Maisy the VR headset. What happened next was remarkable.

"So, Maisy, are they working?" he asked.

"Yeah, I can see your microphone and I can see that you're smiling. And I can see the buttons on your shirt," Maisy replied in astonishment.

"Take a look at the audience," Kelly instructed. "Can you see them all?"

"Yeah, they're waving. I can see there's a lady in the front with a red jacket. The guy next to her is wearing stripes. Oh my god it's so amazing!"

Maisy broke down crying, prompting Kelly and the sold-out audience to follow suit. Then, once Maisy gathered herself, Kelly presented a reading sample from *Harry Potter and the Sorcerer's Stone*. Maisy read it with ease. She hadn't been able to read for years, but regained her ability with the help of VR. The video clip went viral after being posted by the BBC.[4]

Another company called IrisVision also developed a sight augmentation headset.[5] In a 2019 peer-reviewed study using the IrisVision device, researchers from Johns Hopkins found that it improved both reading and visual information processing.[6] The FDA-cleared system is now used by thousands of patients across the world and is offered by major academic medical centers.

Then there's Marcus, the patient who used VR to help recover from his stroke. Here, too, VR is making an impact in the real world. There are over seventy trials testing the benefits of VR for stroke rehabilitation. Although some programs work better than others, meta-analysis reveals that VR improves outcomes when used to augment traditional therapy.[7] In essence, VR offers an elaborate version of V. S. Ramachandran's mirror therapy that we discussed back in Chapter 1. By flipping left and right limbs in VR and convincing the brain that it's moving a paralyzed body part, virtual therapy enables the brain to rebuild damaged neural networks. The science of VR neurorehabilitation has progressed beyond academics. The Swiss company MindMaze obtained FDA clearance in 2017 for its digital mirror therapy program.[8] Now, with the aid of commercially available virtual rehab systems like MindMaze, physical therapists can prescribe exact movements within highly controlled virtual environments. Other startup companies, such as Penumbra and Neuro Rehab VR, are also working to expand the use of VR to overcome brain injuries.

Virtual gyms are also becoming a reality. Although Ramone is a fictional character who used VR to help recover from his heart attack, there is nothing imaginary about virtual reality pushing people to their limits in real reality.[9] Trainers, physical therapists, and rehab specialists are beginning to leverage the unique advantages of training in virtual environments. VR can surround people in motivating scenes, promote proper technique through motion tracking, customize precise range of motion parameters, and allow objective feedback to monitor progress. An innovative company out of Boise, Idaho, called Black Box VR, developed what they call "the world's first full-fitness virtual reality gym experience."[10] Their motto: "Your body is the controller."

As VR gyms become more popular, they will not only serve the walking well but also assist people who are less physically abled. Investigators in Poland, for example, are using VR to reduce falls among the elderly. Research shows that training seniors in supervised virtual gyms can improve stamina, strength, and balance.[11] In Queen's University Belfast, another team is testing VR for people with advanced Parkinson's disease and gait abnormalities.[12] Patients wear a VR headset and see footprints on the ground in a pattern designed to optimize ambulation. The researchers found that interactive VR significantly improves gait performance. Our own team at Cedars-Sinai is evaluating the popular game *Beat Saber* as a tool for physical therapy among patients with arthritis; it's the same game I described for Ramone that involves slicing digital cubes with neon sabers. In a 2018 randomized trial from the University of Kent, researchers confirmed that exercising in VR leads to less pain, a lower perception of effort, and prolonged time to exhaustion compared to a non-VR group.[13] These results are inspiring more doctors to explore VR physical therapy for their patients. Karuna Labs, a San Francisco startup focused on VR rehab, developed a series of evidence-based programs to manage physical impairment from stroke, lower back pain, neuropathic pain, and other chronic disorders.[14] The company developed a network of Virtual Embodiment Training Providers who offer VR physical therapy in their clinical practice, again emphasizing that virtual medicine is not a sci-fi fantasy—virtualists are out there right now seeing patients.

The fictional story of Omar is also based on real patients who are achieving extraordinary progress using immersive therapeutics for spinal cord injuries. In 2016, a multinational team from the US, Switzerland, Germany, and Brazil published the first report using VR brain-machine interfaces to restore mobility in severely paralyzed patients.[15] They studied eight people with complete spinal cord injuries who completed multistage rehabilitation including immersive VR training and walking with an EEG-controlled exoskeleton. After twelve months of therapy, all eight patients showed unprecedented evidence of neurological improvement. More recently, scientists in China have employed a similar VR-based exoskeleton to assist with stroke recovery and found similar success.[16] These examples illustrate how VR, when combined with advances in robotics and biosensor technology, can promote dramatic improvements in physical function.

As we've seen throughout *VRx*, virtual reality can also help people improve mental function. In Chapter 2 we saw how VR helps patients to work through depression and anxiety using virtual self-counseling. Now computer scientists are adding artificial intelligence to the mix in the form of virtual humans, like Mother Teresa in the fictional story of Sarah. The Mother Teresa avatar is inspired by a new field of computer science, called affective computing, that uses objective data to sense mood and counter harmful emotions with precisely timed, contextually relevant treatments. At the University of Southern California, for example, Skip Rizzo created a virtual human who interviews patients with PTSD. The system infers patients' emotional state by measuring facial expressions, body gestures, and vocal parameters. In a published study, Rizzo found that Afghanistan war veterans were more willing to reveal PTSD symptoms to the virtual human than to a real human.[17] In Spain, a team of bioengineers created a VR program that both elicits and auto recognizes emotions using brain waves and heart signals.[18] The system is nearly 80 percent accurate at detecting mood. These examples are especially relevant because there is a worldwide shortage of mental health professionals and limited access to care for many people suffering from anxiety and depression. Virtual humans may not be an ideal substitute for real humans, but they may be better than nothing. In some cases, as Rizzo showed, patients may even prefer the virtual humans who seemingly listen without judgment yet respond in the right way, at the right time.

So, although my day-in-the-life of a virtualist hasn't yet happened, the evidence shows that it can, and that it should. I can only imagine where the science of immersive therapeutics will take us in ten years, but we needn't wait a decade to enact this vision. Let's address the barriers to making virtual medicine an everyday reality.

The waiting room of Attune Health, a medical clinic on the edge of Beverly Hills, is an immersive therapeutic unto itself. Patients wait for their doctor while listening to ethereal music that blends with the sound of water flowing down a stone wall into a pebbly pool by the front desk. On the opposite wall there is a massive photograph of the Los Angeles skyline coming to life under a rising sun. The furniture is modern and sleek, but comfortable. It looks and feels more like a W Hotel than a doctor's office.

Most patients at Attune Health are there because of a rheumatic disease, such as arthritis, lupus, or an inflamed back. But the clinic's medical director, Dr. Swamy Venuturupalli, realized long ago that being a great rheumatologist means thinking beyond the joints. "I can treat arthritis with a steroid injection or numbing medicine, but that doesn't treat the whole patient," he explained. "Some people may only have minor damage to a joint but still experience severe pain, and others have extensive damage but tolerate it well. There's often a disconnect between how people look on an X-ray and how they feel."

Venuturupalli had been following the literature on therapeutic VR and decided to give it a try in his clinic. The first patient he treated was suffering from arthritis along with tremors from multiple sclerosis, a relapsing condition of the central nervous system. He had been struggling to find the best treatments to manage her pain and thought VR might help. "What amazed me," he said, "was not only that VR immediately reduced her pain but also that her tremor, which was pronounced, nearly disappeared while in the VR. When she finally came out twenty minutes later, she felt calm and relaxed. I noticed her hand wasn't shaking and pointed that out to her. She looked at her hands and couldn't believe it. Right then, she realized that her mind has some control over her body. The VR didn't cure her MS, but it definitely made her feel better and gave her back some control, if even for just a little while."

Having witnessed the benefits of VR, Venuturupalli decided to offer the technology to more of his patients. He built a special room in his clinic to administer mind-body treatments like VR, complete with plush couches, a refrigerator full of healthy snacks, dim lights, and a quiet environment away from the bustling of the main work areas. "Now I offer VR as an adjunct to traditional therapies. I might still inject a joint with steroids, but then I'll also administer VR. By addressing both mind and body we have a better chance of making a difference."

Attune Health is one of a growing number of clinics using VR in everyday practice, but virtualists like Venuturupalli are still few and far between. I ask Venuturupalli why more doctors aren't offering VR.

"For many, they just don't know VR even exists. But when I tell colleagues about my experiences using VR and how it works, they all seem to get it. It's not that doctors are afraid; it's just that they just haven't heard of it. They're not sure how it works or where to get the equipment or how to administer the treatments. I think half the battle is just getting the word out."

This first barrier to scaling virtual medicine—educating doctors about the new science of immersive therapeutics—is probably the most tractable. As chair of the education committee for the American College of Rheumatology (ACR), Venuturupalli has worked to incorporate VR into the curriculum of major academic meetings. Now there's at least one lecture per year on immersive therapeutics when the ACR holds its international rheumatology conference. I was fortunate to deliver a keynote talk at the 2018 meeting. The room was packed with several hundred doctors curious to learn more. Our annual Virtual Medicine conference at Cedars-Sinai has also sold out year over year, and our team members travel to a growing number of medical conferences around the world to share what we've learned.

Another accelerant for expanding use of VR is the growing enthusiasm among the newest generation of doctors. Young doctors are not only more knowledgeable than older physicians about technology in general, but they're also the first generation to use VR as part of their medical training. Several prominent medical schools are now substituting VR in anatomy labs instead of cadaveric dissections, prompting students to learn foundational knowledge through the portal of a VR headset.[19] Beyond anatomy, VR is touching nearly every aspect of medical education, from surgical simulations to practicing interviews with patient avatars to rehearsing emergency situations in the safety of a virtual environment. Students can practice complex orthopedic surgeries until they get it right using a program developed by the company Osso VR. A research study proved that students who trained with the software performed better on real knee surgeries compared to a group not exposed to virtual training.[20] Companies like Anima Res, Confideo, Health Scholars, Oxford Medical Simulation, Giblib, and Virti allow students to do things such as interview a virtual patient, practice dousing a fire that erupts in an operating room, or restart a patient's failing heart. As more students use VR to scale steep learning curves faster, they are becoming even more interested in VR and willing to consider it for other aspects of healthcare.

Beyond the barrier of low awareness among doctors is another obstacle to VR adoption: lack of payment. If doctors don't get paid for administering VR, then it will be difficult to scale the technology beyond research centers and motivated clinics like Attune Health. Are insurance companies willing to reimburse immersive therapeutics?

For Dr. Howard Gurr, the answer is yes. Gurr, a psychologist in Long Island, is among a small handful of virtualists in the greater New York area. He practices general psychology but specializes in VR exposure therapy for anxiety and phobias. Gurr uses the same system as Les Posen, the Aussie psychologist profiled in Chapter 5 who treats flight phobias. But Gurr extends his therapy to address all manner of phobias, ranging from fear of spiders to fear of driving over bridges. "I'm the only one in my community offering VR," Gurr said, "and there is no shortage of interest among patients. I'm not really sure why there's so few of us because VR works and it's covered by insurance." VR phobia therapy is a reimbursable service that falls under the covered category of exposure therapy.

Why, then, aren't more psychologists using VR in their practice if it's so effective, sought after by patients, and reimbursable? Gurr's answer is the same as Venuturupalli's: "Because most of my colleagues don't know about it." I expect we will hear this refrain less often as doctors learn about the availability and reimbursement potential for VR, not only for psychotherapy but also for VR physical therapy, which is also covered by insurance.

But insurance does not yet cover VR for pain management, which is surprising since it's the most widely used application of therapeutic VR and is currently offered by several hundred hospitals around the world. In the absence of reimbursement, most hospitals directly pay for VR programs hoping it will save costs by reducing the need for medications and their costly side effects, improve patient satisfaction, or reduce hospital length of stay.

To help insurance companies and healthcare payers understand the potential return on investment of VR pain management, our team published a cost-effectiveness analysis on using VR in the hospital. We performed health economic modeling that accounted for costs related to program implementation, potential savings from decreases in opioid usage and time in the hospital, and effects on patient satisfaction scores that are tied to federal reimbursement for healthcare services.[21]

We found that using VR is very likely to be cost-effective with an average savings of around $100 per patient. Although that's a relatively small positive return, VR could pay substantial dividends if this value were multiplied over thousands of patients per year in a busy hospital. If you consider all the expensive resources that insurance companies cover, like paying for multimillion-dollar robots to perform surgery or using hemodialysis machines for patients at the very end of their life, then buying inexpensive headsets and hiring a few virtualists seems like a low-cost intervention. And if it works while saving money at the same time, then why shouldn't insurers pay for it?

In the meantime, short of insurance coverage, many hospitals are turning to philanthropy to help deliver VR to their patients in need. At Cedars-Sinai, our team was fortunate to receive support from the Marc and Sheri Rapaport Fund for Digital Health Sciences and Precision Health, which allows us to offer VR to many patients without relying on insurance coverage. Pediatric hospitals are also benefiting from major philanthropic support. In 2018, The Walt Disney Company announced a five-year global commitment of $100 million to reimagine the patient and family experience in pediatric hospitals.[22] Disney leveraged its massive team of design experts, called Imagineers, to rethink how immersive technologies can brighten the lives of sick kids by creating a warmer, more personal atmosphere for healing. The company worked with the Starlight Children's Foundation and Stanford University to include VR within its hospital program and is now offering the technology to children's hospitals around the globe. I was fortunate to be an advisor for the program and learned, firsthand, how a company famous for creating joy can focus its expertise on delighting patients in ways few in healthcare know how.

When I think back to my graduation day from medical school, on that beautiful Manhattan afternoon in June 1998—on the stage of Carnegie Hall, no less—I never imagined that I'd one day advise Disney about how to employ immersive therapeutics in a hospital. I never thought that I would prescribe scuba diving excursions to manage IBS, treat hypertension by sending people into their own body to watch salt erode their heart, or transport a hospitalized patient to his favorite park without him leaving the room. I could not imagine using a computer program to combat the opioid epidemic, mainly because I hadn't even heard of the opioid epidemic. I had not experienced departing my physical body and passively observing its lifeless shell from above; nor had I contemplated how such a curious experience might teach me something about dying. I didn't know that I would come face-to-face with an abusive partner in a close-quartered virtual apartment, or how that encounter would fortify my empathy for victims of domestic violence. None of this crossed my mind on that fine spring day when I recited the Hippocratic oath, received my diploma, and donned the forest green robe of a physician.

So much has changed since then: There are hundreds of new medicines; cancer treatments are far more precise; surgery is less invasive and safer; hepatitis C is now curable; people with HIV can live normal lives. These are just a handful of medical revolutions since my graduation.

But when I think about my everyday practice now, the biggest change since I graduated, by far, is the computerization of medicine. When I started as a medical intern at Cedars-Sinai Medical Center in July 1998, I wrote all my notes by hand. If I needed a patient chart, I had to go find it, and that sometimes required a scavenger hunt. I could not always read other doctors' handwriting, and I'm guessing others couldn't read mine. If I wanted to review a chest X-ray, then I had to trudge over to the imaging department, find a radiologist, and rifle through a stack of films to locate the one I needed. Now, after the 2010 Affordable Care Act poured $30 billion into health informatics, every hospital in the United States has an electronic health record. Every note is computerized, every lab value digitized, and every pharmacy order electronically signed. If I need to view an X-ray, I just open my computer and pull up the image.

Beyond advances in electronic recordkeeping, medicine has also fundamentally changed with the emergence of digital health. The idea behind digital health is that we can use smartphones, wearable biosensors like a Fitbit or Apple Watch, and artificial intelligence programs—none of which existed at scale in 1998—to guide health decisions and improve patient outcomes in ways never before possible. When I was an intern, my diabetic patients kept a written log of their daily glucose readings. Now a smartphone app automatically monitors sugar levels and reminds patients when to take their insulin. In 1998, if one of my patients needed to undergo a sleep study, she would spend the night wired up in a lab surrounded by cameras and one-way mirrors and then told to sleep. Now, I can check her Fitbit app and view detailed information about how she's sleeping at home. Digital health is changing everything.[23]

But of all the digital gizmos and gadgets I've encountered so far, it's virtual reality that has commanded my attention. VR is a technology unlike any other in medicine. Whereas the electronic health record requires doctors to spend more time staring at screens than facing their own patients, VR compels doctors to confront the inner lives of their patients and engage in dialogue that might not otherwise occur. It allows doctors to see the world through their patients' eyes rather than directing their gaze to an ever-growing collection of data streams and spreadsheets. It obliges doctors to acknowledge that mind and body both matter for health.

Now, when I encounter diagnostic code Z91.410 in a patient's electronic health record—an alphanumeric that dispassionately maps to "adult physical abuse, domestic"—I imagine that man yelling at me in the virtual simulator. I pause and wonder what my patient had to endure.

Now, when the computer screen displays G30.9, meaning "Alzheimer's disease, unspecified," I think about the child deep inside the patient's mind. I wonder if we can awaken that child with memories of a forgotten past.

When I walked out of Carnegie Hall in 1998 with my diploma, I knew a lot. I knew that hypertension was caused by high vascular resistance. I knew all about the stages of labor and delivery. I knew that people with depression could benefit by changing serotonin levels, or that people with schizophrenia could experience fewer hallucinations by altering dopamine in the brain.

But I didn't know that high blood pressure could respond to a sermon by a pastor. I didn't know that for some women, the pain of childbirth could be lessened by breathing life into a tree. I hadn't a clue that people with depression could rehabilitate through swapping bodies with Sigmund Freud, or that ultraresistant schizophrenia could benefit from a trialogue between therapist, patient, and the patient's inner voice.

I haven't forgotten what I learned in medical school; that knowledge has served me every day since I graduated. But VR has taught me new lessons. It's caused me to think differently about medicine.

More than that, thinking about VR has caused me to think differently about myself. Mel Slater taught me that dying need not be tragic, and that insight caused me to fear death just a little bit less. V. S. Ramachandran and Henrik Ehrsson revealed that my physical sense of self can be easily manipulated, and that assured perceptions of the world—like my location in space and time—might be less certain than I thought. Diane Gromala showed me how VR helps us understand the ways in which the inner world, "the enormous universe within," as she calls it, can be nudged to improve physical and emotional well-being. And Michitaka Hirose demonstrated how primal drives, like the desire to eat, can be instantly modified through digital sleight of hand because "reality," he said, "is in your mind."

As I reflect on these stories and lessons from the book, I keep returning to Hirose's concise summary of his research: *reality is in your mind.*

What does that mean? And what are the implications for virtual medicine? For me, the answer lies in one of my favorite poems, "I Wandered Lonely as a Cloud," by William Wordsworth. As you read these stanzas, try to imagine the vivid scene in your mind's eye:

I wandered lonely as a cloud
That floats on high o'er vales and hills,
When all at once I saw a crowd,
A host, of golden daffodils;
Beside the lake, beneath the trees,
Fluttering and dancing in the breeze.

Continuous as the stars that shine
And twinkle on the milky way,
They stretched in never-ending line
Along the margin of a bay:
Ten thousand saw I at a glance,
Tossing their heads in sprightly dance.

The waves beside them danced; but they
Out-did the sparkling waves in glee:
A poet could not but be gay,
In such a jocund company:
I gazed—and gazed—but little thought
What wealth the show to me had brought:

For oft, when on my couch I lie
In vacant or in pensive mood,
They flash upon that inward eye

Which is the bliss of solitude;
And then my heart with pleasure fills,
And dances with the daffodils.

Can you imagine wandering upon that scene? Can you envision the lake, and the trees, and the daffodils? Can you hear them fluttering in the breeze? Can you hold your imagination long enough to achieve a sense of peace and calm?

If you can experience something about that scene (and most everyone can if they try), then you are living in a virtual reality. That lake isn't real. Those daffodils aren't real. But if you imagine the landscape long enough, and with enough conviction, then it feels real. Reality is in your mind.

We are all living in a virtual reality, almost all of the time. That voice in your head reading these words? Nobody else can hear it. Only you can hear yourself talking to your . . . self. That childhood memory? Only you can see it. That song you can't get out of your head? Only you can hear it. That dream you had last night? Only you experienced it. Virtual reality is part of the human experience.

You can go anywhere in your mind's eye. You can see anything and be anybody. You can construct realities that bear little or no resemblance to your physical environment. Wordsworth closed his eyes to blackness only to reveal ten thousand daffodils. In a mere flash upon the inward eye, he summoned the bliss of solitude. Right now, you can close your eyes and recall fond memories, see close friends, and remember your favorite meals. If you so please, and given the right state of mind and body, you can fill your heart with pleasure.

But not everyone has the same state of mind and body. Not everyone is a Buddhist monk with supernatural abilities to escape reality. Not everyone is healthy enough to entrain their mind without the constant distraction of pain, or discomfort, or a ruminating inner voice. A patient suffering from cancer may struggle to clear enough headspace to imagine a tranquil escape. Someone with post-traumatic stress may be unable to purge memories of a dark past. Our minds are equally able to create ominous virtual realities as they are to project healthy inner worlds. And given all we've learned about the connections between mind and body, our virtual realities can fill our heart with pleasure, as Wordsworth wrote, or wreck our body with pain.

The big idea of virtual medicine is that it leverages our power to imagine when we need it the most. VR modifies our reality in ways that may be hard to accomplish in times of great vulnerability and distress. By carefully adjusting our virtual reality when we are sick, we can affect our physical reality for the better. VR does this by radically changing our perspective of the world. We can imagine being somewhere fantastical and healing. We can practice being the person we want to become. We can see ourselves from beyond and regard ourselves in a new light. We can empathize with ourselves and with others. We can confront our inner voice. We can transform our minds drastically and immediately, and when effective, forge healthy cognitions that last long after the headsets are removed. We already have these abilities within us. VR just makes it easier when times are hard.

When I jumped off that virtual building in 2014 I had never before experienced such an emotionally evocative technology. Plummeting fifty stories to my imagined death was terrifying. But it forced me to wonder: if VR could make people feel bad, then maybe it could also make them feel good. Maybe we could leverage one of the greatest concerns about VR—that it might become like a mind-altering, addictive substance—and flip it on its head by using VR to alter consciousness for the better. Maybe VR could show people that their mind has some governance over their body, and just knowing that—just embodying that knowledge deeply and meaningfully—could help them fight pain, promote cognitive flow, strengthen self-identity, or restore mind-body connections. Maybe VR could alter our perception of the world in a way that, if used thoughtfully and carefully, could improve lives.

In his 1932 dystopian novel *Brave New World*, Aldous Huxley predicted a dark form of mind-controlling VR. He imagined a society programmed like Pavlovian dogs to live pain-free, happy lives through technology and pharmacology. But I have a more beneficent view of how VR will improve human health. I am more inspired by the original source of Huxley's title, which is this stanza from Shakespeare's *The Tempest*:

O wonder!
How many goodly creatures are there here!
How beauteous mankind is! O brave new world,
That has such people in't.

—William Shakespeare, *The Tempest*, act 5, scene 1

When used in the right way, in the right people, and at the right time, VR brings wonder and beauty to mankind. If nothing else, it offers joy. And joy is good. We should leverage that like crazy.

Acknowledgments

When I was in fifth grade, my class was divided into three groups: A, B, and C. Group A was a small group reserved for the smart kids. The teachers never said that, but we all knew it. Group B was the largest group of kids. They were all fine students, but not quite Group A material. Then there was Group C. I was a Group C kid. To this day, I define my educational origin as a kid at the bottom. By any objective standard, I was not a good student. Writing was a challenge. Math didn't come easy. I scored in the 8th percentile on a standardized exam. I remember filling out the multiple-choice grid like I was playing a game of Battleship. Turns out that correct answers don't typically align in exact diagonal or vertical stripes. It's fair to say that my eleven-year-old self could not have imagined writing anything of substance, much less a book. I certainly wouldn't have imagined becoming a doctor, or a professor, or a researcher.

Thankfully, our school principal, Reveta Bowers, saw something in me. She spent time getting to know me and figured out that I was living in a sort of virtual reality in my head. When it came time for middle school, Reveta called up Dave Velasquez, the director of admissions at the local college prep school, and asked him to ignore my test scores, overlook my grades, and let me in. He did. I was so inspired by their confidence that I awoke from my educational slumber and dedicated myself to becoming a Group A student. This book might not have been possible without them. I also want to acknowledge key mentors along the way, including Edward McCatty, for teaching me how to think critically; Daniel Dennett, for critiquing how I think; C. S. Pitchumoni, for teaching me what to think about; and Josh Ofman, for revealing how thoughts can make a difference. Thanks also to my postdoctoral mentors at UCLA, including Gareth Dulai, Ian Gralnek, Emeran Mayer, and Roger Bolus, for teaching me how to ask and answer scientific questions.

This book also would not be possible without Shlomo Melmed, the dean of our faculty at Cedars-Sinai, who, on a whim, sent me an email in 2014 about a new technology called virtual reality. Dr. Melmed knew I was interested in technology and heard that VR might be useful for managing pain, so he sent me the info. A half decade later, we've treated over three thousand people at Cedars-Sinai using VR, published numerous clinical trials, launched an annual VR conference, and received NIH funding for our research. All from one email. I also want to thank the leadership at Cedars-Sinai, including Tom Priselac and Scott Weingarten, for inviting me into the organization and cultivating an academic environment that supports and values meaningful innovation.

Special thanks also to Josh Sackman and Matthew Stoudt for forcing me to jump off a fifty-story building in 2014. It was their software that created my first VR experience. Together with Walter Greenleaf, Josh and Matthew introduced me to VR and for that I will be forever grateful.

Writing this book required that I cover broad swaths of healthcare. At various times I felt like an honorary psychiatrist, neuroscientist, geriatrician, cardiologist, rheumatologist, pain specialist, and pediatrician. I was fortunate that many of my colleagues were willing to review parts of the book to ensure I didn't stray too far off the evidentiary rails. Special thanks to Brandon Birckhead, Itai Danovitch, Adam Gazzaley, Rafael Grossmann, Les Posen, Skip Rizzo, Mel Slater, and Melissa Wong for reading early drafts of the book. I'd also like to thank all the scientists, clinicians, and developers who provided information for the book, including Justin Barad, Kate Donovan, Alexandre Dumais, Molly Easterlin, Scott Gorman, Diane Gromala, Howard Gurr, Ted Jones, Ramon Oliva, Kyle Rand, Arfa Rehman, Nanea Reeves, Mavi Sanchez-Vives, and Swamy Venuturupalli.

I am especially indebted to all the patients who allowed me to tell their stories. Deep thanks go to Richard Breton, Danielle Collins, Harmon Clarke, Tom Norris, Robert Jester, and Erin Martucci. I also wish to thank all the patients at Cedars-Sinai who have trusted us with their care and have been willing to try VR as part of their treatment.

This book would not exist were it not for the support of my research team, graduate students, and VR research colleagues at Cedars-Sinai. At risk of leaving someone out, I wish to thank Michael Albert, Fadi Alhatem, Chris Almario, Jeanne Black, Michelle Chen, Bernice Coleman, Kruttika Dabke, Francis Dailey, Sean Delshad, Taylor Dupuy, Sam Eberlein, Garth Fuller, Becca Gale, John Garlich, Waguih IsHak, Mariko Ishimori, Alma Jusufagic, Carine Khalil, Mayra Lopez, Milton Little, Xiaoyu Liu, Ben Noah, Kathy Oka, Shervin Rabizadeh, Brad Rosen, Kelvin Sauls, Jennifer Soares, Vartan Tashjian, Mechauna Thierry, Joe Tu, Mani Vahedi, Welmoed van Deen, Mark Vrahas, and Kyung Yu. Thanks also to members of our communications team at Cedars-Sinai for their advocacy, including Soshea Liebler, Duke Helfand, and Marni Usheroff.

As a research scientist I couldn't get very far without funding. Our lab has been extremely fortunate to receive generous research grants and philanthropic support. Special thanks to Marc and Sheri Rapaport for establishing their Fund for Digital Health Sciences and Precision Health at Cedars-Sinai, which supported much of our early VR research. Thanks also to Art Ochoa for working with the Rapaports to establish their fund. Further credit goes to AppliedVR, Bayer, The Mayday Fund, Northwest Mutual Life Foundation, Samsung Electronics, the Hearst Foundation, HP, Traveler's Insurance, The Walt Disney Company, and the National Institutes of Health for their support of our VR program at Cedars-Sinai.

Books don't get published without talented agents and editors. Thanks to Jim Levine for his willingness to read an amateur book proposal from an untested author and then, to my astonishment, immediately jump aboard. Jim has been a true advocate of this project from the start. Eric Henney at Basic Books did a spectacular job editing the manuscript. He always asked the tough questions, forced me to dig deeper than I knew how, and gently guided me to write in English rather than in medicalese. If Eric had run away after reading my first draft chapter, well, I wouldn't have blamed him. But he stuck with me and never failed to deliver timely and valid critiques. This book is so much better because of Eric. Thanks also to Mike van Mantgem for his expert copyediting.

My parents raised me to be curious, to always ask questions, and to have enough grit to finish this book. In 1986, during my eighth grade final exams, they gave me a card that said, "Do the best you can. Nobody can ask more, and you won't be satisfied with anything less." It's a platitude, yet to me the card has always felt deeply meaningful. I kept it with me throughout my adult life and now my daughter has it on her desk; I looked at it often while writing this book. Thanks also to my mom for reading every chapter of the manuscript and providing useful feedback throughout.

I dedicate this book to my wife, Tracy, and my children, Kaelen and Shane. Without them I'd be lost and confused. With them I am whole and sustained. Tracy is the most selfless and kind person I know. She put up with me working late and disappearing for hours to write this book, yet never once made a point to mention my untimely absences. As a writing professor, she read early drafts of the manuscript and always provided gentle yet precise guidance when my writing went astray. I also want to thank my daughter for lending her hands to model Ramachandran's mirror box (first photograph in Chapter 1), and my son for his undying enthusiasm for my VR research. More importantly, I want to thank both of them for putting up with my absences while writing this book, and for just being awesome kids. I can only say I'm terribly lucky to have my family; they make living in real reality an ever-present joy.

Notes and References

Introduction: A Leap of Faith

1. Jaron Lanier, *Dawn of the New Everything: A Journey Through Virtual Reality* (London: Penguin Random House, 2017), 56.

2. "Virtual and Augmented Reality: Understanding the Race for the Next Computing Platform," Goldman Sachs, January 13, 2016, www.goldmansachs.com/insights /pages/technology-driving-innovation-folder/virtual-and-augmented-reality/report .pdf.

3. The term "digiceutical" refers to a new class of digital treatments that includes biosensors, smartphone applications, and nondrug immersive therapeutics like VR. The US Food and Drug Administration now considers digiceuticals to be a legitimate form of therapy and regulates their approval.

4. The term "empathy machine" is often used to describe the perspective-taking capabilities of VR. It is generally credited to Chris Milk, who gave a TED Talk: "How Virtual Reality Can Create the Ultimate Empathy Machine," filmed March 2015, www.ted.com /talks/chris_milk_how_virtual_reality_can_create_the_ultimate_empathy_machine.

Chapter 1: The Second Time I Died

1. Daniel Dennett has written many books over his illustrious career, but the volume that most influenced me is *Consciousness Explained* (Boston: Little, Brown, 1991).

2. Hilary Putnam, *Reason, Truth and History* (Cambridge: Cambridge University Press, 1981), 1–21.

3. René Descartes originated the earliest version of the brain-in-a-vat argument in his 1641 treatise, *Meditations on First Philosophy*. There, he described the Evil Demon argument, where he pondered whether he could ever disprove the possibility that life is served up as an illusion from a deceptive devil. He concluded that he could not know, for sure, whether or not he was being duped. Descartes could only know that he existed ("I think, therefore I am," he said famously). Some might wonder if VR is the modern Evil Demon imposing unsavory realities upon unsuspecting souls, something we explore in this book.

4. V. S. Ramachandran and D. Rogers-Ramachandran, "Synaesthesia in Phantom Limbs Induced with Mirrors," *Proceedings of the Royal Society London* 263 (1996): 377–386.

5. Ramachandran and Ramachandran, "Synaesthesia in Phantom Limbs," 377–386.

6. Henrik Ehrsson, "What if We Could Leave Our Body and Have a New One?," March 28, 2016, TEDxGöteborg, Gothenburg, Sweden, video, www.youtube.com /watch?v=ZEhXX47PRvw. In this TED Talk, Ehrsson begins by posing his early life questions about embodiment, and he then describes how he dedicated his career to scientifically investigating the answers. If you want to learn more about Ehrsson's work and how it is forcing us to confront our sense of self, read Ed Yong, "Out-of-Body Experience: Master of Illusion," *Nature* 480 (2011): 168–170.

7. M. Botvinick and J. Cohen, "Rubber Hand 'Feels' Touch That Eyes See," *Nature* 391 (1998): 756.

8. H. H. Ehrsson, N. P. Holmes, and R. E. Passingham, "Touching a Rubber Hand: Feeling of Body Ownership Is Associated with Activity in Multisensory Brain Areas," *Journal of Neuroscience* 25 (2005): 10564–10573.

9. H. H. Ehrsson, K. Weich, N. Weiskopf, et al., "Threatening a Rubber Hand That You Feel Is Yours Elicits a Cortical Anxiety Response," *Proceedings of the National Academy of Sciences of the United States of America* 104 (2007): 9828–9833. You can go online and watch videos of people reacting to their rubber hand being attacked, some with a fork, some with a knife, some with a hammer; it's a convincing response. Here is an example: www.youtube.com/watch?v=sxwn1w7MJvk.

10. V. I. Petkova and H. H. Ehrsson, "If I Were You: Perceptual Illusion of Body Swapping," *PLoS ONE* 3 (2008): e3832.

11. Petkova and Ehrsson, "If I Were You," e3832.

12. B. Van der Hoort, A. Guterstam, and H. H. Ehrsson, "Being Barbie: The Size of One's Own Body Determines the Perceived Size of the World," *PLoS ONE* 6 (2011): e20195.

13. BeAnotherLab, "The Machine to Be Another," www.beanotherlab.org/home /work/tmtba.

14. A. Souppouris, "Virtual Reality Made Me Believe I Was Someone Else," *The Verge*, March 24, 2014, www.theverge.com/2014/3/24/5526694/virtual-reality-made -me-believe-i-was-someone-else.

15. Ehrsson, "What if We Could Leave Our Body."

16. S. Schnall, J. R. Zadra, and D. R. Proffitt, "Direct Evidence for the Economy of Action: Glucose and the Perception of Geographical Slant," *Perception* 39 (2010): 464–482.

17. We call this the brain-gut axis. For an authoritative guide on the linkage between mind and microbiome, read *The Mind-Gut Connection* by Emeran Mayer, MD. I was fortunate to work with Dr. Mayer as a postdoctoral student at UCLA, where I participated in his pioneering research evaluating brain-gut connections in digestive diseases. I cover his work in Chapter 3 because it helps explain why VR can manage abdominal pain in conditions like irritable bowel syndrome.

18. K. Tillisch, J. Labus, L. Kilpatrick, et al., "Consumption of Fermented Milk Product with Probiotic Modulates Brain Activity," *Gastroenterology* 144 (2013): 1394–1401.

19. There are many sources to learn about the theory of embodied cognition. I am most influenced by the work of Antonio Damasio, a professor of neuroscience at the University of Southern California who has performed foundational research explaining the connections between mind and body. Damasio has evolved his model over hundreds of citations, but for a concise and authoritative review I recommend this citation: A. Damasio and G. B. Carvalho, "The Nature of Feelings: Evolutionary and Neurobiological Origins," *Nature Reviews Neuroscience* 14 (2013): 143–152. For a lay review of his theory of consciousness, I recommend his book *Self Comes to Mind: Constructing the Conscious Brain* (New York: First Vintage Books, 2010).

20. Alan Jasanoff, *The Biological Mind: How Brain, Body and Environment Collaborate to Make Us Who We Are* (New York: Basic Books, 2018).

21. Michael Pollan, *How to Change Your Mind: What the New Science of Psychedelics Teaches Us About Consciousness, Dying, Addiction, Depression, and Transcendence* (New York: Penguin Random House, 2018), 285.

22. P. Bourdin, I. Barberia, R. Oliva, et al., "A Virtual Out-of-Body Experience Reduces Fear of Death," *PLoS ONE* 12 (2017): e0169343.

23. I. Barberia, R. Oliva, P. Bourdin, and M. Slater, "Virtual Mortality and Near-Death Experience After a Prolonged Exposure in a Shared Virtual Reality May Lead to Positive Life-Attitude Changes," *PLoS ONE* 13 (2018): e0203358. This video shows scenes from the virtual island and the out-of-body experience: www.youtube.com/watch?v=C_eTXCqJObA&feature=youtu.be.

Chapter 2: The Self Blends

1. Steven Kotler and Jamie Wheal, *Stealing Fire: How Silicon Valley, the Navy SEALs, and Maverick Scientists Are Revolutionizing the Way We Live and Work* (New York: HarperCollins, 2017), 28–32.

2. Kotler and Wheal, *Stealing Fire*, 31–32.

3. Mihaly Csikszentmihalyi, *Flow: The Psychology of Optimal Experience* (New York: Harper & Row, 1990).

4. Kotler and Wheal, *Stealing Fire*, 111.

5. Mark R. Leary, *The Curse of the Self: Self-Awareness, Egotism, and the Quality of Human Life* (New York: Oxford University Press, 2004), 8.

6. The term "highway hypnosis" was first credited to an article written by G. W. Williams, titled appropriately enough, "Highway Hypnosis," *International Journal of Clinical and Experimental Hypnosis* 103 (1963): 143–151. But the observation that drivers tune out for long stretches of road dates back to the 1920s.

7. Jan Null, CCM, "Heatstroke Deaths of Children in Vehicles," Department of Meteorology and Climate Science, San Jose State University, www.noheatstroke.org.

8. Adam Gazzaley and Larry D. Rosen, *The Distracted Mind: Ancient Brains in a High-Tech World* (Cambridge, MA: MIT Press, 2016).

9. Gazzaley and Rosen, *Distracted Mind*, 9.

10. M. E. Raichle, A. M. LacLeod, A. Z. Snyder, et al., "A Default Mode of Brain Function," *Proceedings of the National Academy of Sciences USA* 98 (2001): 676–682.

11. Michael Pollan, *How to Change Your Mind: What the New Science of Psychedelics Teaches Us About Consciousness, Dying, Addiction, Depression, and Transcendence* (New York: Penguin Random House, 2018), 302.

12. M. A. Killingsworth and D. T. Gilbert, "A Wandering Mind Is an Unhappy Mind," *Science* 12 (2010): 932.

13. A. Dietrich, "Functional Neuroanatomy of Altered States of Consciousness: The Transient Hypofrontality Hypothesis," *Consciousness and Cognition* 12 (2003): 231–256.

14. This figure of forty-four thousand hours of meditative practice is based on a scientific report of Buddhist monks performed by Richard J. Davidson and Antoine Lutz, "Buddha's Brain: Neuroplasticity and Meditation," *IEEE Signal Processing Magazine* 25 (2008): 174–176.

15. Kotler and Wheal, *Stealing Fire*, 36.

16. Z. Josipovic, "Neural Correlates of Nondual Awareness in Meditation," *Annals of the New York Academy of Sciences* 1307 (2014): 9–18. Also see M. Kozhevnikov, O. Louchakova, Z. Josipovic, et al., "The Enhancement of Visuospatial Processing Efficiency Through Buddhist Deity Meditation," *Psychological Science* 20 (2009): 645–653.

17. For an excellent review of the history of LSD's synthesis at Sandoz Lab and its subsequent history, read Michael Pollan, *How to Change Your Mind: What the New Science of Psychedelics Teaches Us About Consciousness, Dying, Addiction, Depression, and Transcendence* (New York: Penguin Random House, 2018).

18. Pollan, *How to Change Your Mind*, 263.

19. R. L. Carhart-Harris, D. Erritzoe, T. Williams, et al., "Neural Correlates of the Psychedelic State as Determined by fMRI Studies with Psilocybin," *Proceedings of the National Academy of Sciences USA* 109 (2012): 2138–2143.

20. M. W. Johnson, A. Garcia-Romeu, and R. R. Griffiths, "Long-Term Follow-Up of Psilocybin-Facilitated Smoking Cessation," *American Journal of Drug and Alcohol Abuse* 43 (2017): 55–60.

21. R. R. Griffiths, M. W. Johnson, M. A. Carducci, et al., "Psilocybin Produces Substantial and Sustained Decreases in Depression and Anxiety in Patients with Life-Threatening Cancer: A Randomized Double-Blind Trial," *Journal of Psychopharmacology* 30 (2016): 1181–1197.

22. R. R. Griffiths, W. A. Richards, U. McCann, et al., "Psilocybin Can Occasion Mystical-Type Experiences Having Substantial and Sustained Personal Meaning and Spiritual Significance," *Psychopharmacology* 187 (2006): 268–283.

23. K. Suzuki, W. Roseboom, D. J. Schwartzman, et al., "A Deep-Dream Virtual Reality Platform for Studying Altered Perceptual Phenomenology," *International Journal of Scientific Reports* 22 (2017): 15982.

24. It may be hard to imagine this fantastical scene of people walking around a university campus with dog heads and bells. Here's a video of the experiment: www.youtube.com/watch?v=TlMBnCrZZYY.

25. A. Dittrich, "The Standardized Psychometric Assessment of Altered States of Consciousness (ASCs) in Humans," *Pharmacopsychiatry* 31 (1998): 80–84.

26. Watch this video to learn more about *Bravemind* VR exposure therapy for PTSD: https://vimeo.com/100452938.

27. Rizzo and his team have published over ten studies evaluating the effectiveness of his VR exposure therapy. Here is a selection of studies: A. Rizzo, T. D. Parsons, B. Lange, et al., "Virtual Reality Goes to War: A Brief Review of the Future of Military

Behavioral Healthcare," *Journal of Clinical Psychology in Medical Settings* 18 (2011): 176–187; A. Rizzo, J. G. Buckwalter, B. John, et al., "STRIVE: Stress Resilience in Virtual Environments: A Pre-deployment VR System for Training Emotional Coping Skills and Assessing Chronic and Acute Stress Responses," *Studies in Health Technology and Informatics* 173 (2012): 379–385; R. N. McLay, K. Graap, J. Spira, et al., "Development and Testing of Virtual Reality Exposure Therapy for Post-Traumatic Stress Disorder in Active Duty Service Members Who Served in Iraq and Afghanistan," *Military Medicine* 177 (2012): 635–642; A. Rizzo and R. Shilling, "Clinical Virtual Reality Tools to Advance the Prevention, Assessment, and Treatment of PTSD," *European Journal of Psychotraumatology* 16 (2017): 1414560.

28. B. O. Rothbaum, A. Rizzo, and J. Difede, "Virtual Reality Exposure Therapy for Combat-Related Posttraumatic Stress Disorder," *Annals of the New York Academy of Sciences* 1208 (2010): 126–132.

29. K. B. Highland, M. Costanzo, T. Jovanovic, et al., "Catecholamine Responses to Virtual Combat: Implications for Post-Traumatic Stress and Dimensions of Functioning," *Frontiers in Psychology: Quantitative Psychology and Measurement* 6 (2015): 256, 1–7. And see S. D. Norrholm, T. Jovanovic, M. Gerardi, et al., "Baseline Psychophysiological and Cortisol Reactivity as a Predictor of PTSD Treatment Outcome in Virtual Reality Exposure Therapy," *Behaviour Research and Therapy* 82 (2016): 28–37.

30. M. J. Roy, M. E. Costanzo, J. R. Blair, et al., "Compelling Evidence That Exposure Therapy for PTSD Normalizes Brain Function," *Studies in Health Technology and Informatics* 199 (2014): 61–65.

31. There are now over one hundred studies evaluating VR exposure therapy across anxiety disorders. In this note, I have collected examples of what I consider to be some of the most important studies. For arachnophobia: S. Minns, A. Levihn-Coon, E. Carl, et al., "Immersive 3D Exposure-Based Treatment for Spider Fear: A Randomized Controlled Trial," *Journal of Anxiety Disorders* 61 (2019): 37–44. For agoraphobia: E. Malbos, R. M. Rapee, and M. Kavakli, "A Controlled Study of Agoraphobia and the Independent Effect of Virtual Reality Exposure Therapy," *Australian & New Zealand Journal of Psychiatry* 47 (2013): 160–168. Notably, the literature on VR for agoraphobia has been more conflicted than for other anxiety conditions. Here is an example of a study where VR was not superior: K. Meyerbroeker, N. Morina, G. A. Kerkhof, et al., "Virtual Reality Exposure Therapy Does Not Provide Any Additional Value in Agoraphobic Patients: A Randomized Controlled Trial," *Psychotherapy and Psychosomatics* 82 (2013): 170–176. For fear of heights: T. Donker, I. Cornelisz, C. van Klaveren, et al., "Effectiveness of Self-Guided App-Based Virtual Reality Cognitive Behavior Therapy for Acrophobia: A Randomized Clinical Trial," *JAMA Psychiatry* (2019): 682–690. For fear of flying: B. O. Rothbaum, L. Hodges, P. L. Anderson, et al., "Twelve-Month Follow-Up of Virtual Reality and Standard Exposure Therapies for the Fear of Flying," *Journal of Consulting and Clinical Psychology* 70 (2002): 428–432. See also B. K. Wiederhold, D. P. Jang, R. G. Gevirtz, et al., "The Treatment of Fear of Flying: A Controlled Study of Imaginal and Virtual Reality Graded Exposure Therapy," *IEEE Transactions on Information Technology in Biomedicine* 6 (2002): 218–223. For generalized anxiety disorder: A. Gorini, F. Pallavicini, D. Algeri, et al., "Virtual Reality in the Treatment of Generalized Anxiety Disorders," *Studies in Health Technology and Informatics* 154 (2010): 39–43. See also

M. V. Navarro-Haro, M. Modrego-Alarcón, H. G. Hoffman, et al., "Evaluation of a Mindfulness-Based Intervention with and Without Virtual Reality Dialectical Behavior Therapy(®) Mindfulness Skills Training for the Treatment of Generalized Anxiety Disorder in Primary Care: A Pilot Study," *Frontiers in Psychology* 10 (2019): 55. For panic disorder: M. A. Pérez-Ara, S. Quero, C. Botella, et al., "Virtual Reality Interoceptive Exposure for the Treatment of Panic Disorder and Agoraphobia," *Studies in Health Technology Informatics* 154 (2010): 77–81. For social anxiety: S. Bouchard, S. Dumoulin, G. Robillard, et al., "Virtual Reality Compared with In Vivo Exposure in the Treatment of Social Anxiety Disorder: A Three-Arm Randomised Controlled Trial," *British Journal of Psychiatry* 210 (2017): 276–283.

32. E. Carl, A. T. Stein, A. Levihn-Coon, et al., "Virtual Reality Exposure Therapy for Anxiety and Related Disorders: A Meta-Analysis of Randomized Controlled Trials," *Journal of Anxiety Disorders* 61 (2019): 27–36.

33. Caroline J. Falconer, Mel Slater, Aitor Rovira, et al., "Embodying Compassion: A Virtual Reality Paradigm for Overcoming Excessive Self-Criticism," *PLoS ONE* 9 (2014): e111933.

34. Sofia A. Osimo, Rodrigo Pizarro Lozano, Bernhard Spanlang, et al., "Conversations Between Self and Self as Sigmund Freud—A Virtual Body Ownership Paradigm for Self-Counselling," *Scientific Reports* 10 (2015): 13899.

35. Osimo et al., "Conversations Between Self."

36. Osimo et al., "Conversations Between Self."

Chapter 3: Creating a Distraction

1. Erin's story is based on several interviews I conducted with her in 2018 and 2019. In addition, she told her story as part of a patient panel at the 2018 Virtual Medicine Conference at Cedars-Sinai; filmed with her permission on March 29, 2018, in Los Angeles, California, www.youtube.com/watch?v=GKZWWBQj_W4.

2. You can view the original "invisible gorilla" video here: www.youtube.com/watch?v=vJG698U2Mvo. For more information, read *The Invisible Gorilla: How Our Intuition Deceives Us* by Christopher Chabris and Daniel Simons (New York: Random House, 2009). It's one of my all-time favorite books.

3. Here is the second invisible gorilla video, in case you've already seen the first video: www.youtube.com/watch?v=IGQmdoK_ZfY.

4. T. Drew, M. L. H. Vo, and K. Wolfe, "The Invisible Gorilla Strikes Again: Sustained Inattentional Blindness in Expert Observers," *Psychological Science* 24 (2013): 1848–1853.

5. The distinction between distraction and interruption is well described in Adam Gazzaley and Larry D. Rosen, *The Distracted Mind: Ancient Brains in a High-Tech World* (Cambridge, MA: MIT Press, 2016), chapter 1.

6. Gazzaley and Rosen, *Distracted Mind*, 9.

7. Linda Stone, "Continuous Partial Attention," https://lindastone.net/qa/continuous-partial-attention.

8. W. C. Clapp, M. T. Rubens, and A. Gazzaley, "Mechanisms of Working Memory Disruption by External Interference," *Cerebral Cortex* 20 (2009): 859–872.

9. Gazzaley and Rosen, *Distracted Mind*, 57.

10. Denise Grady, "The Vision Thing: Mainly in the Brain," *Discover Magazine*, June 1993.

11. Gazzaley and Rosen, *Distracted Mind*, 34–36.

12. S. Üstün, E. H. Kale, and M. Çiçek, "Neural Networks for Time Perception and Working Memory," *Frontiers in Human Neuroscience* 24 (2017): 83; H. Y. Lee and E. L. Yang, "Exploring the Effects of Working Memory on Time Perception in Attention Deficit Hyperactivity Disorder," *Psychological Reports* 122 (2019): 23–35.

13. Clapp, Rubens, and Gazzaley, "Mechanisms of Working Memory Disruption by External Interference," 859–872; W. C. Clapp and A. Gazzaley, "Distinct Mechanisms for the Impact of Distraction and Interruption on Working Memory in Aging," *Neurobiology of Aging* 33 (2012): 134–148.

14. N. JahaniShoorab, S. E. Zagami, A. Nahvi, et al., "The Effect of Virtual Reality on Pain in Primiparity Women During Episiotomy Repair: A Randomized Clinical Trial," *Iranian Journal of Medical Sciences* 40 (2015): 219–224. Of note, VR time acceleration is not limited to obstetrics. Research has also demonstrated the effect among patients receiving chemotherapy. See S. M. Schneider and L. E. Hood, "Virtual Reality: A Distraction Intervention for Chemotherapy," *Oncology Nursing Forum* 34 (2007): 39–46.

15. D. Frey, M. Bauer, C. Bell, et al., "Virtual Reality Analgesia in Labor: The VRAIL Pilot Study—A Preliminary Randomized Controlled Trial Suggesting Benefit of Immersive Virtual Reality Analgesia in Unmedicated Laboring Women," *Anesthesia & Analgesia* 128 (2019): e93–e96.

16. M. S. Wong, B. M. R. Spiegel, and K. D. Gregory, "Virtual Reality Reduces Pain in Laboring Women: A Randomized Controlled Trial," presented at the 2020 Society for Maternal-Fetal Medicine Meeting, Grapevine, Texas. Full manuscript in peer review at the time of publication.

17. R. Melzack and P. D. Wall, "Pain Mechanisms: A New Theory," *Science* 150 (1965): 971–979.

18. For a discussion about Descartes's original concept of pain and how it fits into Melzack and Wall's modern theory, read R. Melzack and J. Katz, "Pain," *WIREs Cognitive Science* 4 (2013): 1–15.

19. *SnowWorld* is among the most famous and evidence-based therapeutic VR software programs ever created. Hunter Hoffman and David Patterson at the University of Washington are credited not only for developing and validating *SnowWorld*, but more generally, for developing the concept of VR analgesia. Here are some of their key references, among others not shown for lack of space: H. G. Hoffman, D. R. Patterson, and G. J. Carrougher, "Use of Virtual Reality for Adjunctive Treatment of Adult Burn Pain During Physical Therapy: A Controlled Study," *Clinical Journal of Pain* 16 (2000): 244–250; H. G. Hoffman, S. R. Sharar, B. Coda, et al., "Manipulating Presence Influences the Magnitude of Virtual Reality Analgesia," *Pain* 111 (2004): 162–168; H. G. Hoffman, D. R. Patterson, E. Seibel, et al., "Virtual Reality Pain Control During Burn Wound Debridement in the Hydrotank," *Clinical Journal of Pain* 24 (2008): 299–304; H. G. Hoffman, G. T. Chambers, W. J. Meyer III, et al., "Virtual Reality as an Adjunctive Non-Pharmacologic Analgesic for Acute Burn Pain During Medical Procedures," *Annals of Behavioral Medicine* 41 (2011): 183–191.

20. Y. S. Schmitt, H. G. Hoffman, D. K. Blough, et al., "A Randomized, Controlled Trial of Immersive Virtual Reality Analgesia, During Physical Therapy for Pediatric Burns," *Burns* 37 (2011): 61–68.

21. H. G. Hoffman, T. L. Richards, T. Van Oostrom, et al., "The Analgesic Effects of Opioids and Immersive Virtual Reality Distraction: Evidence from Subjective and Functional Brain Imaging Assessments," *Anesthesia and Analgesia* 105 (2007): 1776–1783. For more information on the effects of VR analgesia on the brain, see H. G. Hoffman, T. L. Richards, A. R. Bills, et al., "Using FMRI to Study the Neural Correlates of Virtual Reality Analgesia," *CNS Spectrums* 11 (2006): 45–51.

22. There are now hundreds of studies testing VR analgesia across a wide range of acute conditions. In this note I provide some key examples. For dental procedures: M. D. Wiederhold, K. Gao, and B. K. Wiederhold, "Clinical Use of Virtual Reality Distraction System to Reduce Anxiety and Pain in Dental Procedures," *Cyberpsychology, Behavior, and Social Networking* 17 (2014): 359–365; P. Indovina, D. Barone, L. Gallo, et al., "Virtual Reality as a Distraction Intervention to Relieve Pain and Distress During Medical Procedures: A Comprehensive Literature Review," *Clinical Journal of Pain* 34 (2018): 858–877. For spinal taps: S. Sander Wint, D. Eshelman, J. Steele, et al., "Effects of Distraction Using Virtual Reality Glasses During Lumbar Punctures in Adolescents with Cancer," *Oncology Nursing Forum* 29 (2002): E8–E15. For urological procedures: J. Y. Moon, J. Shin, J. Chung, et al., "Virtual Reality Distraction During Endoscopic Urologic Surgery Under Spinal Anesthesia: A Randomized Controlled Trial," *Journal of Clinical Medicine* 20 (2018). For colonoscopy: T. Lembo, L. Fitzgerald, K. Matin, et al., "Audio and Visual Stimulation Reduced Patient Discomfort During Screening Flexible Sigmoidoscopy," *American Journal of Gastroenterology* 93 (1998): 1113–1116; D. W. Lee, A. C. Chan, S. K. Wong, et al., "Can Visual Distraction Decrease the Dose of Patient-Controlled Sedation Required During Colonoscopy? A Prospective Randomized Controlled Trial," *Endoscopy* 36 (2004): 197–201. For chemotherapy: Susan M. Schneider and Linda E. Hood, "Virtual Reality: A Distraction Intervention for Chemotherapy," *Oncology Nursing Forum* 34 (2007): 39–46. For intravenous needle sticks there are over one hundred studies. Here are two papers summarizing three randomized trials: E. Chan, M. Hovenden, E. Ramage, et al., "Virtual Reality for Pediatric Needle Procedural Pain: Two Randomized Clinical Trials," *Journal of Pediatrics* 209 (2019): 160–167; S. Dumoulin, S. Bouchard, J. Ellis, et al., "A Randomized Controlled Trial of the Use of Virtual Reality for Needle-Related Procedures in Children and Adolescents in the Emergency Department," *Games for Health Journal* (2019).

23. V. Leibovici, F. Magora, S. Cohen, et al., "Effects of Virtual Reality Immersion and Audiovisual Distraction Techniques for Patients with Pruritus," *Pain Research and Management* 4 (2009): 283–286.

24. E. Chan, S. Foster, R. Sambell, and P. Leong, "Clinical Efficacy of Virtual Reality for Acute Procedural Pain Management: A Systematic Review and Meta-Analysis," *PLoS ONE* 13 (2018): e0200987.

25. H. R. Berthoud and W. L. Neuhuber, "Functional and Chemical Anatomy of the Afferent Vagal System," *Autonomic Neuroscience* 85 (2000): 1–17.

26. The origin of the term "second brain" in relation to the human gastrointestinal system is attributed to Michael Gershon, a renowned gastrointestinal physiologist from Columbia University in New York. For more, read Michael Gershon, *The Second Brain:*

A Groundbreaking New Understanding of Nervous Disorders of the Stomach and Intestine (New York: HarperCollins, 1998).

27. For an authoritative analysis of how our "second brain" influences our "first brain," read Emeran Mayer, *The Mind-Gut Connection: How the Hidden Conversation Within Our Bodies Impacts Our Mood, Our Choices, and Our Overall Health* (New York: HarperCollins, 2016).

28. For information about the impact of the Sandanista revolution on subsequent abdominal pain and IBS, see this reference: D. Wurzelmann, R. Pena, L. Cortes, et al., "Positive Association Between Traumatic War Experiences in the Sandinista Revolution and Subsequent IBS: A Population-Based Study in Nicaragua," *Digestive Disease Week* Abstract 299 (2008). See also S. Becker-Dreps, D. Morgan, R. Peña, et al., "Association Between Intimate Partner Violence and Irritable Bowel Syndrome: A Population-Based Study in Nicaragua," *Violence Against Women* (2010): 832–845.

29. R. M. Lovell and A. C. Ford, "Global Prevalence of and Risk Factors for Irritable Bowel Syndrome: A Meta-Analysis," *Clinical Gastroenterology and Hepatology* 10 (2012): 712–721.

30. Although there are controversies about the causes of IBS, most scientists agree it is a problem of the "brain-gut axis." For a full-throated defense of this theory, read Mayer, *Mind-Gut Connection*.

31. Mayer, *Mind-Gut Connection*.

32. A. C. Ford, B. E. Lacy, L. A. Harris, et al., "Effect of Antidepressants and Psychological Therapies in Irritable Bowel Syndrome: An Updated Systematic Review and Meta-Analysis," *American Journal of Gastroenterology* 114 (2019): 21–39.

33. V. Tashjian, S. Mosadeghi, M. Reid, et al., "Virtual Reality Reduces Abdominal Pain in Hospitalized Patients: Results of a Controlled Trial," *Gastroenterology* 152 (2017): S115.

34. J. Pamment and J. E. Aspell, "Putting Pain out of Mind with an 'Out of Body' Illusion," *European Journal of Pain* 2 (2017): 334–342.

Chapter 4: Becoming Whole

1. For more details about Richard Breton's story, refer to this detailed, peer-reviewed case report published by Breton in partnership with Alexandre Dumais and his research team: L. Dellazizzo, O. Percie du Sert, S. Potvin, R. Breton, et al., "Avatar Therapy for Persistent Auditory Verbal Hallucinations: A Case Report of a Peer Research Assistant on His Path Toward Recovery," *Psychosis* (2018): 1–7.

2. J. McGrath, S. Saha, D. Chant, et al., "Schizophrenia: A Concise Overview of Incidence, Prevalence, and Mortality," *Epidemiologic Reviews* 30 (2008): 67–76.

3. M. L. Hu, X. F. Zong, J. J. Mann, et al., "A Review of the Functional and Anatomical Default Mode Network in Schizophrenia," *Neuroscience Bulletin* 33 (2017): 73–84.

4. H. Lee, D. K. Lee, K. Park, et al., "Default Mode Network Connectivity Is Associated with Long-Term Clinical Outcome in Patients with Schizophrenia," *NeuroImage: Clinical* 22 (2019): 101805.

5. Hu et al., "Default Mode Network in Schizophrenia," 73–84.

6. A. Aleman and F. Larøi, "Insights into Hallucinations in Schizophrenia: Novel Treatment Approaches," *Expert Review of Neurotherapeutics* 11 (2011): 1007–1015.

7. M. van der Gaag, L. R. Valmaggia, and F. Smit, "The Effects of Individually Tailored Formulation-Based Cognitive Behavioural Therapy in Auditory Hallucinations and Delusions: A Meta-Analysis," *Schizophrenia Research* 156 (2014): 30–37.

8. J. Leff, G. Williams, M. A. Huckvale, et al., "Computer-Assisted Therapy for Medication-Resistant Auditory Hallucinations: Proof-of-Concept Study," *British Journal of Psychiatry* 202 (2013): 428–433.

9. P. Berman, "Julian Leff: Changing the Face of Schizophrenia Treatment," *Lancet Psychiatry* 4 (2018): 302.

10. T. K. J. Craig, M. Rus-Calafell, T. Ward, et al., "AVATAR Therapy for Auditory Verbal Hallucinations in People with Psychosis: A Single-Blind, Randomised Controlled Trial," *Lancet Psychiatry* 5 (2018): 31–40.

11. O. Percie du Sert, S. Potvin, O. Lipp, L. Dellazizzo, M. Laurelli, R. Breton, P. Lalonde, K. Phraxayavong, K. O'Connor, J. Pelletier, T. Boukhalfi, P. Renaud, and A. Dumais, "Virtual Reality Therapy for Refractory Auditory Verbal Hallucinations in Schizophrenia: A Pilot Clinical Trial," *Schizophrenia Research* 197 (2018): 176–181. I've opted to list all the authors of this article to highlight that Richard Breton, the patient discussed in Chapter 4, is also an author in this peer-reviewed study.

12. Jacob Cohen, *Statistical Power Analysis for the Behavioral Science* (London: Academic Press, 1977).

13. Du Sert et al., "Virtual Reality Therapy."

14. Du Sert et al., "Virtual Reality Therapy."

15. E. Granholm and P. D. Harvey, "Social Skills Training for Negative Symptoms of Schizophrenia," *Schizophrenia Bulletin* 44 (2018): 472–474.

16. L. H. Adery, M. Ichinose, L. J. Torregrossa, et al., "The Acceptability and Feasibility of a Novel Virtual Reality Based Social Skills Training Game for Schizophrenia: Preliminary Findings," *Psychiatry Research* 270 (2018): 496–502.

17. Adery et al., "Social Skills Training Game for Schizophrenia."

18. M. Rus-Calafell, P. Garety, E. Sason, et al., "Virtual Reality in the Assessment and Treatment of Psychosis: A Systematic Review of Its Utility, Acceptability and Effectiveness," *Psychological Medicine* 48 (2018): 362–391.

19. Mar Rus-Calafell was quoted in an article by Joshua Hwang, "The Cutting Edge of Schizophrenia Research: VR as Treatment for Psychosis," *Psychiatry Advisor*, April 30, 2018.

20. Marcus Raichle was quoted in an article by Matt Danzico, "Brains of Buddhist Monks Scanned in Meditation Study," BBC News, April 24, 2011. Although the article is about Buddhist monks, it covers the default mode network and includes comments by Raichle regarding the DMN and its abnormalities in Alzheimer's dementia.

21. M. D. Greicius, G. Srivastava, A. L. Reiss, et al., "Default-Mode Network Activity Distinguishes Alzheimer's Disease from Healthy Aging: Evidence from Functional MRI," *Proceedings of the National Academy of Sciences of the USA* 101 (2004): 4637–4642.

22. B. Woods, L. O'Philbin, E. M. Farrell, et al., "Reminiscence Therapy for Dementia," *Cochrane Database of Systematic Reviews* 3 (2018): CD001120.

23. Ben Tinker, "'Dementia Village' Inspires New Care," CNN, December 27, 2013, www.cnn.com/2013/07/11/world/europe/wus-holland-dementia-village

/index.html. There is an accompanying documentary on the website featuring Dr. Sanjay Gupta that offers a deep dive into the facility and its operations.

24. Jennifer Wolff, "Re-Created 1950s City Helps to Ease Dementia's Grasp: Glenner Town Square Offers Comfort for Those with Cognitive Decline," *AARP Bulletin*, December 7, 2018.

25. "Virtual Reality Opens World of Possibilities for Seniors," CBS News, September 1, 2016, www.cbsnews.com/news/virtual-reality-rendever-mit-company-helps-seniors-physical-limitations-travel-world.

26. Reed Hayes is quoted by journalist Katheleen Conti, "MIT Startup Lets Seniors Enter the World of Virtual Reality," *Boston Globe*, May 12, 2016.

27. Based on a phone interview conducted with Kyle Rand, CEO of Rendever, on April 26, 2019.

28. Scott Gorman is quoted by journalist Benjamin Powers, "How Virtual Reality Can Help Fight Dementia: Recreated Memories," *The Daily Beast*, November 2, 2018 (last modified April 30, 2019), www.thedailybeast.com/how-virtual-reality-can-help-fight-dementia.

29. Xueyang (Charles) Lin, "Designing Virtual Reality (VR) Experience for Older Adults and Determin[ing] Its Impact on Their Overall Well-Being" (master's thesis, MIT, June 2017).

30. C. C. Hsieh, P. S. Lin, W. C. Hsu, et al., "The Effectiveness of a Virtual Reality–Based Tai Chi Exercise on Cognitive and Physical Function in Older Adults with Cognitive Impairment," *Dementia and Geriatric Cognitive Disorders* 46 (2018): 358–370.

31. A. R. Sakhare, V. Yang, J. Stradford, et al., "Cycling and Spatial Navigation in an Enriched, Immersive 3D Virtual Park Environment: A Feasibility Study in Younger and Older Adults," *Frontiers in Aging Neuroscience* (2019): 218.

32. S. Arlati, V. Colombo, D. Spoladore, et al., "A Social Virtual Reality–Based Application for the Physical and Cognitive Training of the Elderly at Home," *Sensors* (Basel) 19 (2019).

33. S. Zygouris, K. Ntovas, D. Giakoumis, et al., "A Preliminary Study on the Feasibility of Using a Virtual Reality Cognitive Training Application for Remote Detection of Mild Cognitive Impairment," *Journal of Alzheimer's Disease* 56 (2017): 619–627.

34. For more on Nanthia Suthana's work, see this article and video by Elaine Schmidt, "Neuroscientist Harnesses the Power of Virtual Reality to Unlock the Mysteries of Memory," UCLA, August 30, 2017, http://newsroom.ucla.edu/stories/neuroscientist-harnesses-the-power-of-virtual-reality-to-unlock-the-mysteries-of-memory. Also see Nicco Reggente, Joey K.-Y. Essoe, Zahra M. Aghajan, et al., "Enhancing the Ecological Validity of fMRI Memory Research Using Virtual Reality," *Frontiers in Neuroscience* 12 (2018): 408.

35. For more information on *Sea Hero Quest*, visit this website: https://www.telekom.com/en/corporate-responsibility/corporate-responsibility/sea-hero-quest-game-for-good-587134.

Chapter 5: Mind the Gap

1. For more on the "sensory immersion vessel," watch Adam Gazzaley's lecture from the 2019 Virtual Medicine Conference at Cedars-Sinai, filmed with his permission

on March 27, 2019, in Los Angeles, California. Video (discussion about immersion vessel occurs at 14:30 into the video): www.youtube.com/watch?v=0zVLdTIu_lc.

2. For more on the principles of closed-loop systems, read Adam Gazzaley's essay, "The Cognition Crisis," *Medium*, July 9, 2018, https://medium.com/s/futurehuman/the-cognition-crisis-a1482e889fcb.

3. A. Gorini, F. Pallavicini, D. Algeri, et al., "Virtual Reality in the Treatment of Generalized Anxiety Disorders," *Studies in Health Technology Informatics* 154 (2010): 39–43.

4. Jeff Tarrant, Jeremy Viczko, and Hannah Cope, "Virtual Reality for Anxiety Reduction Demonstrated by Quantitative EEG: A Pilot Study," *Frontiers in Psychology* 9 (2018): 1280.

5. For more on interoceptive accuracy and interoceptive awareness, see Sarah N. Garfinkel, Anil K. Seth, Adam B. Barrett, et al., "Knowing Your Own Heart: Distinguishing Interoceptive Accuracy from Interoceptive Awareness," *Biological Psychology* 104 (2015): 65–74.

6. For a thorough discussion about the science of interoception, including its impact on life experiences, read an outstanding and authoritative review authored by Noga Arikha, "The Interoceptive Turn," Aeon, June 17, 2019, https://aeon.co/essays/the-interoceptive-turn-is-maturing-as-a-rich-science-of-selfhood.

7. D. Di Lernia, S. Serino, N. Polli, et al., "Interoceptive Axes Dissociation in Anorexia Nervosa: A Single Case Study with Follow Up Post-Recovery Assessment," *Frontiers in Psychology* 9 (2019): 2488.xxfdi.

8. Di Lernia et al., "Anorexia Nervosa."

9. G. Riva and A. Dakanalis, "Altered Processing and Integration of Multisensory Bodily Representations and Signals in Eating Disorders: A Possible Path Toward the Understanding of Their Underlying Causes," *Frontiers in Human Neuroscience* 12 (2018): 49.

10. A. Keizer, A. van Elburg, R. Helms, et al., "A Virtual Reality Full Body Illusion Improves Body Image Disturbance in Anorexia Nervosa," *PLoS ONE* 11 (2016): e0163921.

11. Keizer et al., "Body Image Disturbance in Anorexia Nervosa."

12. S. Serino, N. Polli, and G. Riva, "From Avatars to Body Swapping: The Use of Virtual Reality for Assessing and Treating Body-Size Distortion in Individuals with Anorexia," *Journal of Clinical Psychology* 75 (2019): 313–322.

13. D. Clus, M. E. Larsen, C. Lemey, et al., "The Use of Virtual Reality in Patients with Eating Disorders: Systematic Review," *Journal of Medical Internet Research* 20 (2018): e157.

14. Di Lernia et al., "Anorexia Nervosa."

15. G. Riva and A. Dakanalis, "Altered Processing and Integration of Multisensory Bodily Representations and Signals in Eating Disorders: A Possible Path Toward the Understanding of Their Underlying Causes," *Frontiers in Human Neuroscience* 12 (2018): 49.

16. S. Serino, F. Scarpina, A. Keizer, et al., "A Novel Technique for Improving Bodily Experience in a Non-Operable Super–Super Obesity Case," *Frontiers in Psychology* 7 (2016): 837.

17. G. M. Manzoni, G. L. Cesa, M. Bacchetta, et al., "Virtual Reality–Enhanced Cognitive-Behavioral Therapy for Morbid Obesity: A Randomized Controlled Study with 1 Year Follow-Up," *Cyberpsychology, Behavior, and Social Networking* 19 (2016): 134–140.

18. T. Narumi, Y. Ban, T. Kajinami, et al., "Augmented Perception of Satiety: Controlling Food Consumption by Changing Apparent Size of Food with Augmented Reality," *Proceedings of the SIGCHI Conference on Human Factors in Computing Systems* (2012): 109–118.

19. T. Narumi, S. Nishizaka, T. Kajinami, et al., "MetaCookie+," *IEEE Virtual Reality Conference* (2011): 265–266.

20. *The Week* staff, "The 'Diet Glasses' That Trick You into Eating Less," *The Week*, June 5, 2012.

Chapter 6: The Virtualist

1. World Health Organization, "What Is the WHO Definition of Health?," www.who.int/about/who-we-are/frequently-asked-questions.

2. G. L. Engel, "The Need for a New Model: A Challenge for Biomedicine," *Science* 196 (1977): 129–136.

3. This program is called the Patient Reported Outcome Measurement Information System, or PROMIS for short. For more information about PROMIS and other health surveys, visit www.healthmeasures.net. My research lab created the PROMIS questionnaires for digestive health; we use these surveys in our own clinic to monitor whether our treatments are actually helping.

4. S. Mosadeghi, M. Reid, B. Martinez, et al., "Feasibility of an Immersive Virtual Reality Intervention for Hospitalized Patients: An Observational Cohort Study," *JMIR Mental Health* 3 (2016): e28.

5. Like any medical device, VR headsets have potential to spread infection if they are not carefully sanitized between uses. In our hospital, we clean the headsets using a strict protocol to help reduce risk of infectivity. Technicians wipe down fabric surfaces with a one-step disinfectant called Virex, and then scrub the plastic housing using Sani-Wipes. We use an alcohol-based cleaner on the glass lenses and also apply a new foam backing for each patient that fits around the headset and serves as a buffer between the user's face and the headset; this reduces direct contact with the device. In following this protocol at Cedars-Sinai, we have not documented spread of infection with VR headsets. We previously used a fitted head cap (called a bouffant) to reduce direct contact with the hair and scalp, but have since determined that extra step is low yield if the device is properly cleaned and the foam backing is replaced between each use. Another approach is to use UV light, which bathes the device with bug-blasting energy. A company called Cleanbox created a UV box specifically designed to clean VR headsets. This approach is probably easier and more reliable than hand-cleaning headsets; we are now exploring both options. If your hospital is using VR, then be sure to ask how frequently the devices are cleaned and with what technique. If there is any uncertainty, then you could request to watch the headset be cleaned in person. Be sure to ask whether a new foam backing was affixed prior to use. If your hospital does not use unique foam backing for each patient, then find out more about how they reduce infection risk.

6. Mosadeghi et al., "Virtual Reality Intervention."

7. Mosadeghi et al., "Virtual Reality Intervention."

8. V. C. Tashjian, S. Mosadeghi, A. R. Howard, et al., "Virtual Reality for Management of Pain in Hospitalized Patients: Results of a Controlled Trial," *JMIR Mental Health* 4 (2017): e9.

9. In medicine, we commonly compare treatments using a statistic called the number needed to treat, or NNT. The NNT is a standard metric used to compare the benefits of different therapies across healthcare. It turns out that a 25 percent difference in response translates into an NNT of 4. In other words, for every four patients who received VR instead of watching the relaxation video, there was one additional person who achieved a clinically meaningful response. By way of comparison, the NNT of powerful opioid medicines like morphine is around 5 to 10, or more, depending on the study (a lower NNT is better). More in Chapter 6.

10. B. Spiegel, G. Fuller, M. Lopez, et al., "Virtual Reality for Management of Pain in Hospitalized Patients: A Randomized Comparative Effectiveness Trial," *PLoS ONE* 14 (2019): e0219115.

11. For more on Harmon's moving story, watch his keynote lecture from the 2019 Virtual Medicine Conference at Cedars-Sinai, filmed with his permission on March 28, 2019, in Los Angeles, California: www.youtube.com/watch?v=7DM3O8L2wgU.

Chapter 7: Fighting the Opioid Epidemic

1. For a deep dive into the false advertising and scandalous promotion of opioids by Purdue Pharmaceuticals, the manufacturer of OxyContin, read Beth Macy, *Dopesick: Dealers, Doctors, and the Drug Company That Addicted America* (New York: Little, Brown, 2018).

2. James Dahlhamer, Jacqueline Lucas, Carla Zelaya, et al., "Prevalence of Chronic Pain and High-Impact Chronic Pain Among Adults—United States, 2016," *Sensors* (Basel) 67 (2018): 1001–1006.

3. National Institute on Drug Abuse, "Overdose Death Rates," www.drugabuse .gov/related-topics/trends-statistics/overdose-death-rates.

4. A. Shah, C. Hayes, and B. C. Martin, "Characteristics of Initial Prescription Episodes and Likelihood of Long-Term Opioid Use—United States, 2006–2015," *Morbidity and Mortality Weekly Report* 66 (2017): 265–269.

5. W. A. Ray, C. P. Chung, K. T. Murray, et al., "Prescription of Long-Acting Opioids and Mortality in Patients with Chronic Noncancer Pain," *Journal of the American Medical Association* 315 (2016): 2415–2423.

6. For a full account of this multifaceted story, read Martin Booth, *Opium: A History* (New York: St. Martin's Griffin, 1999).

7. The term "opioid" technically refers to these opium-like synthetic compounds. In contrast, "opiates" are drugs naturally derived from the poppy plant, such as heroin, morphine, and codeine. Most people now refer to all of these drugs as "opioids" for short, although there are subtle differences.

8. J. Porter and H. Jick, "Addiction Rare in Patients Treated with Narcotics," *New England Journal of Medicine* 302 (1980): 123.

9. P. T. M. Leung, E. M. Macdonald, I. A. Dhalla, et al., "A 1980 Letter on the Risk of Opioid Addiction," *New England Journal of Medicine* 376 (2017): 2194–2195.

10. For more on the history of the opioid epidemic, including the Joint Commission booklet sponsored by Purdue Pharmaceuticals, read Sonia Moghe, "Opioid History: From 'Wonder Drug' to Abuse Epidemic," CNN, updated October 14, 2016, www.cnn .com/2016/05/12/health/opioid-addiction-history/index.html.

11. Despite the polarization of American politics, one thing all sides seem to agree upon is the need to address the opioid epidemic. The Helping to End Addiction Long-Term (HEAL) initiative is one of many bipartisan efforts to help end the crisis. For more information on HEAL, visit www.nih.gov/research-training/medical -research-initiatives/heal-initiative.

12. For an accessible academic review of acute versus chronic pain and the concept of pain sensitization, read R. Melzack and J. Katz, "Pain," *WIREs Cognitive Science* 4 (2013): 1–15.

13. Melzack and Katz, "Pain," 1.

14. Diane Gromala, "Curative Powers of Wet, Raw Beauty," TEDxAmericanRiviera, December 7, 2011, www.youtube.com/watch?v=cRdarMz--Pw.

15. For more on Gromala's VR research for chronic pain, watch her lecture from the 2019 Virtual Medicine Conference at Cedars-Sinai, "A Mirror for the Soul: How VR Cures by Enabling Self-Awareness," filmed with her permission on March 27, 2019, in Los Angeles, California: www.youtube.com/watch?v=umj7mSRtUsI.

16. D. Gromala, X. Tong, A. Choo, et al., "The Virtual Meditative Walk: Virtual Reality Therapy for Chronic Pain Management" (paper presented at the ACM CHI Conference, Seoul, Republic of Korea, April 18–23, 2015).

17. T. V. Salomons, T. Johnstone, M. Backonja, et al., "Perceived Controllability Modulates the Neural Response to Pain," *Journal of Neuroscience* 24 (2004): 7199–7203.

18. W. Jin, A. Choo, D. Gromala, et al., "A Virtual Reality Game for Chronic Pain Management: A Randomized, Controlled Clinical Study," *Studies in Health Technology and Informatics* 220 (2016): 154–160.

19. H. Sarig-Bahat, P. L. Weiss, and Y. Laufer, "Neck Pain Assessment in a Virtual Environment," *Spine* 35 (2010): E105–112. Also see K. B. Chen, M. E. Sesto, K. Ponto, et al., "Use of Virtual Reality Feedback for Patients with Chronic Neck Pain and Kinesiophobia," *IEEE Transactions on Neural Systems and Rehabilitation Engineering* (2016): 1240–1248.

20. VR has now been used for many different chronic pain conditions. I've collected exemplar studies in this note. For fibromyalgia: J. P. Martín-Martínez, S. Villafaina, D. Collado-Mateo, et al., "Effects of 24-Week Exergame Intervention on Physical Function Under Single- and Dual-Task Conditions in Fibromyalgia: A Randomized Controlled Trial," *Scandinavian Journal of Medicine & Science in Sports* 29 (2019): 1610–1617. For chronic migraine headaches: S. Shiri, U. Feintuch, N. Weiss, et al., "A Virtual Reality System Combined with Biofeedback for Treating Pediatric Chronic Headache—A Pilot Study," *Pain Medicine* 14 (2013): 621–627. For phantom limb pain: J. Dunn, E. Yeo, P. Moghaddampour, et al., "Virtual and Augmented Reality in the Treatment of Phantom Limb Pain: A Literature Review," *NeuroRehabilitation* 40 (2017): 595–601. Notably, in

this review of the literature, the authors concluded that the evidence for VR treatment of phantom limb pain, although promising, is still not extensive enough to support wide-scale adoption, and that further research is needed. For spinal cord injuries: E. Yeo, B. Chau, B. Chi, et al., "Virtual Reality Neurorehabilitation for Mobility in Spinal Cord Injury: A Structured Review," *Innovations in Clinical Neuroscience* 16 (2019): 13–20. For complex regional pain syndrome: A. S. Won, C. A. Tataru, C. M. Cojocaru, et al., "Two Virtual Reality Pilot Studies for the Treatment of Pediatric CRPS," *Pain Medicine* 16 (2015): 1644–1647. See also: C. McCabe, R. Haigh, E. Ring, et al., "A Controlled Pilot Study of the Utility of Mirror Visual Feedback in the Treatment of Complex Regional Pain Syndrome (Type 1)," *Rheumatology* 42 (2003): 97–101.

21. Madison Wade, "Overdose Memorial Christmas Tree Decorated to Remember Lives Lost," 10News, Knoxville, November 29, 2017, www.wbir.com/article/news/local/overdose-memorial-christmas-tree-decorated-to-remember-lives-lost/51-495615167.

22. T. Jones, T. Moore, and J. Choo, "The Impact of Virtual Reality on Chronic Pain," *PLoS ONE* 11 (2016): e0167523.

23. T. Jones, R. Skadberg, and T. Moore, "A Pilot Study of the Impact of Repeated Sessions of Virtual Reality on Chronic Neuropathic Pain," *International Journal of Virtual Reality* 18 (2018): 19–34.

24. For more on how Ted Jones is using VR for chronic pain, watch his lecture from the 2019 Virtual Medicine Conference at Cedars-Sinai, "Battling the Opioid Epidemic with Virtual Reality: Front-Line Experiences from the Clinical Trenches," filmed with his permission on March 27, 2018, in Los Angeles, California: www.youtube.com/watch?v=INjT4JkdZpM.

25. C. E. Rutter, L. M. Dahlquist, and K. E. Weiss, "Sustained Efficacy of Virtual Reality Distraction," *Journal of Pain* 10 (2009): 391–397.

26. H. G. Hoffman, D. R. Patterson, G. J. Carrougher, et al., "Effectiveness of Virtual Reality–Based Pain Control with Multiple Treatments," *Clinical Journal of Pain* 17 (2001): 229–235.

27. H. G. Hoffman, T. L. Richards, T. Van Oostrom, et al., "The Analgesic Effects of Opioids and Immersive Virtual Reality Distraction: Evidence from Subjective and Functional Brain Imaging Assessments," *Anesthesia and Analgesia* 105 (2007): 1776–1783.

28. T. McSherry, M. Atterbury, S. Gartner, et al., "Randomized, Crossover Study of Immersive Virtual Reality to Decrease Opioid Use During Painful Wound Care Procedures in Adults," *Journal of Burn Care & Research* 39 (2018): 278–285.

29. In addition to the studies described in the chapter, another group of investigators at Prince of Wales Hospital, Hong Kong, used VR to distract patients undergoing colonoscopy. They found that using a combination of visual and auditory distraction reduced the need for Propofol, a powerful intravenous sedative, by nearly 40 percent. See D. W. Lee, A. C. Chan, S. K. Wong, et al., "Can Visual Distraction Decrease the Dose of Patient-Controlled Sedation Required During Colonoscopy? A Prospective Randomized Controlled Trial," *Endoscopy* 36 (2004): 197–201.

30. A. C. Williams, C. Eccleston, and S. Morley, "Psychological Therapies for the Management of Chronic Pain (Excluding Headache) in Adults," *Cochrane Database of Systematic Reviews* 11 (2012): CD007407; K. Bernardy, N. Füber, V. Köllner, et al.,

"Efficacy of Cognitive-Behavioral Therapies in Fibromyalgia Syndrome—A Systematic Review and Metaanalysis of Randomized Controlled Trials," *Journal of Rheumatology* 37 (2010): 1991–2005.

31. L. C. Wu, P. W. Weng, C. H. Chen, et al., "Literature Review and Meta-Analysis of Transcutaneous Electrical Nerve Stimulation in Treating Chronic Back Pain," *Regional Anesthesia and Pain Medicine* 43 (2018): 425–433.

Chapter 8: Primum Non Nocere

1. Institute of Medicine (US) Committee on Quality of Health Care in America; L. T. Kohn, J. M. Corrigan, and M. S. Donaldson, editors, "To Err Is Human: Building a Safer Health System," Washington, DC: National Academies Press, 2000.

2. K. Lecroy, "The Lie of Primum Non Nocere," *American Family Physician* 64 (2001): 1942.

3. J. S. Spiegel, "The Ethics of Virtual Reality Technology: Social Hazards and Public Policy Recommendations," *Science and Engineering Ethics* 24 (2018): 1537–1550. As an aside, although there aren't many Spiegels in the academic VR world, I have no relation with this particular Spiegel.

4. For a detailed history of scientific inquiry regarding the human vestibular system, including accomplishments by Duverney, Scarpa, Ewald, and Baranay, read Sapan S. Desai and Anahita Dua, "History of Research in the Vestibular System: A 400-Year-Old Story," *Journal of Anatomy and Physiology* 4 (2014).

5. For more on the threats to scaling the consumer VR business, read Blake J. Harris, *The History of the Future: Oculus, Facebook, and the Revolution That Swept Virtual Reality* (New York: HarperCollins, 2019).

6. N. Dużmańska, P. Strojny, and A. Strojny, "Can Simulator Sickness Be Avoided? A Review on Temporal Aspects of Simulator Sickness," *Frontiers in Psychology* 9 (2018): 2132.

7. Rebecca Searles, "Virtual Reality Can Leave You with an Existential Hangover," *Atlantic*, December 21, 2016.

8. From a post found by Rebecca Searles on MTBS3D.com and linked to in her *Atlantic* article, https://www.mtbs3d.com/phpBB/viewtopic.php?f=140&t=17753 #p130268, August 3, 2008.

9. Tobias van Schneider, "The Post Virtual Reality Sadness," *Medium* (blog), https://medium.com/desk-of-van-schneider/the-post-virtual-reality-sadness-fb4a1ccacae4.

10. K. J. Jáuregui-Renaud, "Vestibular Function and Depersonalization/Derealization Symptoms," *Multisensory Research* (2015).

11. J. A. Bernat, H. M. Ronfeldt, K. S. Calhoun, et al., "Prevalence of Traumatic Events and Peritraumatic Predictors of Posttraumatic Stress Symptoms in a Nonclinical Sample of College Students," *Journal of Traumatic Stress* 11 (1998): 645–664.

12. N. M. Simon, M. H. Pollack, K. S. Tuby, et al., "Dizziness and Panic Disorder: A Review of the Association Between Vestibular Dysfunction and Anxiety," *Annals of Clinical Psychiatry* 10 (1998): 75–80.

13. In addition to the 1998 review by Simon et al. of thirty studies linking vestibular dysfunction to panic disorder, many more studies since that time have evaluated the relationship between the inner ear and psychiatric disorders like panic and anxiety. Here

are a few more recent examples: R. T. Bigelow, Y. R. Semenov, S. du Lac, et al., "Vestibular Vertigo and Comorbid Cognitive and Psychiatric Impairment: The 2008 National Health Interview Survey," *Journal of Neurology, Neurosurgery, and Psychiatry* 87 (2016): 367–372; C. M. Coelho and C. D. Balaban, "Visuo-Vestibular Contributions to Anxiety and Fear," *Neuroscience & Biobehavioral Reviews* 48 (2015): 148–159; Y. Saman, D. E. Bamiou, M. Gleeson, et al., "Interactions Between Stress and Vestibular Compensation—A Review," *Frontiers in Neurology* 3 (2012): 116.

14. F. Aardema, K. O'Connor, S. Côté, et al., "Virtual Reality Induces Dissociation and Lowers Sense of Presence in Objective Reality," *Cyberpsychology, Behavior, and Social Networking* 13 (2010).

15. K. Y. Segovia and J. N. Bailenson, "Virtually True: Children's Acquisition of False Memories in Virtual Reality," *Media Psychology* 12 (2009): 371–393.

16. There are many reports of using therapeutic VR in pediatrics. Here are some examples, starting with VR distraction during needle sticks: A. Dunn, J. Patterson, C. F. Biega, et al., "A Novel Clinician-Orchestrated Virtual Reality Platform for Distraction During Pediatric Intravenous Procedures in Children with Hemophilia: Randomized Controlled Trial," *JMIR Serious Games* 7 (2019): e10902; B. Atzori, H. G. Hoffman, L. Vagnoli, et al., "Virtual Reality Analgesia During Venipuncture in Pediatric Patients with Onco-Hematological Diseases," *Frontiers in Psychology* 9 (2018): 2508. For spinal taps: J. J. Thomas, J. Albietz, and D. Polaner, "Virtual Reality for Lumbar Puncture in a Morbidly Obese Patient with Leukemia," *Paediatric Anaesthesia* 28 (2018): 1059–1060. For dental procedures: B. Atzori, R. Lauro-Grotto, A. Giugni, et al., "Virtual Reality Analgesia for Pediatric Dental Patients," *Frontiers in Psychology* 23 (2018): 2265.

17. A sample of representative studies: M. Maskey, J. Rodgers, V. Grahame, et al., "A Randomised Controlled Feasibility Trial of Immersive Virtual Reality Treatment with Cognitive Behaviour Therapy for Specific Phobias in Young People with Autism Spectrum Disorder," *Journal of Autism and Developmental Disorders* 49 (2019): 1912–1927; R. Chad, S. Emaan, and O. Jillian, "Effect of Virtual Reality Headset for Pediatric Fear and Pain Distraction During Immunization," *Pain Management* 8 (2018): 175–179; S. Shiri, U. Feintuch, N. Weiss, et al., "A Virtual Reality System Combined with Biofeedback for Treating Pediatric Chronic Headache—A Pilot Study," *Pain Medicine* 14 (2013): 621–627; M. R. Golomb, B. C. McDonald, S. J. Warden, et al., "In-Home Virtual Reality Videogame Telerehabilitation in Adolescents with Hemiplegic Cerebral Palsy," *Archives of Physical Medicine and Rehabilitation* 91 (2010): 1–8.e1.

18. Beata Mostafavi, "Harbaugh Fund Helps Mott Patients Virtually Experience the Big House," *Michigan Health*, November 29, 2016.

19. "Virtual Reality: A New Dimension in Medicine," CGTN News, December 31, 2016, https://america.cgtn.com/2016/12/31/virtual-reality-a-new-dimension-in-medicine.

20. Medgadget editors, "Sevo the Dragon Uses Fire Breath to Distract Kids from Getting Anesthesia," *Medgadget*, April 18, 2017, www.medgadget.com/2017/04/sevo-dragon-uses-fire-breath-distract-kids-getting-anesthesia.html. Also see S. Rodriguez, J. H. Tsui, S. Y. Jiang, et al., "Interactive Video Game Built for Mask Induction in Pediatric Patients," *Canadian Journal of Anaesthesia* 64 (2017): 1073–1074.

21. S. N. V. Yuan and H. H. S. Ip, "Using Virtual Reality to Train Emotional and Social Skills in Children with Autism Spectrum Disorder," *London Journal of Primary Care* 19 (2018): 110–112.

22. A. T. Booth, A. I. Buizer, J. Harlaar, et al., "Immediate Effects of Immersive Biofeedback on Gait in Children with Cerebral Palsy," *Archives of Physical Medicine and Rehabilitation* 100 (2019): 598–605.

23. Some notable reads from a vast literature: Margaret Morris, *Left to Our Own Devices: Outsmarting Smart Technology to Reclaim Our Relationships, Health, and Focus* (Boston: MIT Press, 2018); M. D. Griffiths and M. N. O. Davies, "Videogame Addiction: Does It Exist?," in J. Raessens and J. Goldstein, eds., *Handbook of Computer Game Studies* (Boston: MIT Press, 2005), 359–368; M. D. Griffiths and N. Hunt, "Dependence on Computer Game Playing by Adolescents," *Psychological Reports* 82 (1998): 475–480; C. A. Anderson and B. J. Bushman, "Effects of Violent Video Games on Aggressive Behavior, Aggressive Cognition, Aggressive Affect, Physiological Arousal, and Prosocial Behavior: A Meta-Analytic Review of the Scientific Literature," *Psychological Science* 12 (2001): 353–359.

24. Jeremy Bailenson, *Experience on Demand* (New York: W. W. Norton, 2018), 52.

25. Jaron Lanier, *Dawn of the New Everything: A Journey Through Virtual Reality* (London: Penguin Random House, 2017), 54.

26. "Sony Pictures Entertainment Launches Innovation Studios: Dell, Deloitte Digital and Intel Collaborate on New Venture Where Technology Meets Story," press release, June 7, 2018, www.sonypictures.com/corp/press_releases/2018/06_18/060718 _innovationstudios.html. Note that at the time I met with Scot Barbour he was vice president of production for Innovation Studios serving under the studio president, Glenn Gainor. Barbour has since left Innovation Studios, which remains under Gainor's oversight at the time of this writing.

27. Spiegel, "Ethics of Virtual Reality Technology."

28. M. Madary and T. K. Metzinger, "Real Virtuality: A Code of Ethical Conduct: Recommendations for Good Scientific Practice and the Consumers of VR-Technology," *Frontiers in Robotics and AI* 3 (2016), www.frontiersin.org/articles/10.3389 /frobt.2016.00003/full.

29. Daniel Oberhaus, "We're Already Violating Virtual Reality's First Code of Ethics," *Vice*, March 6, 2016, www.vice.com/en_us/article/yp3va5/vr-code-of-ethics.

Chapter 9: The VR Pharmacy

1. The literature on binaural beats is expansive albeit somewhat contradictory. An important study supporting the benefits of binaural beats was published in 2003; it was a randomized trial using binaural beats compared to standard audio with patients about to have surgery. The study revealed that binaural beats were superior for reducing anxiety. Here is the reference: R. Padmanabhan, A. J. Hildreth, and D. Laws, "A Prospective, Randomized, Controlled Study Examining Binaural Beat Audio and Pre-Operative Anxiety in Patients Undergoing General Anaesthesia for Day Case Surgery," *Anaesthesia* 60 (2005): 874–877.

2. J. F. Bridges, A. B. Hauber, D. Marshall, et al., "Conjoint Analysis Applications in Health—A Checklist: A Report of the ISPOR Good Research Practices for Conjoint Analysis Task Force," *Value in Health* (2011): 403–413.

3. *IBD&me* is available for free at www.ibdandme.org.

4. C. V. Almario, M. S. Keller, M. Chen, et al., "Optimizing Selection of Biologics in Inflammatory Bowel Disease: Development of an Online Patient Decision Aid Using Conjoint Analysis," *American Journal of Gastroenterology* (2018): 58–71.

5. M. S. Wong, B. M. Spiegel, and K. D. Gregory, "Virtual Reality Reduces Pain in Laboring Women: A Randomized Controlled Trial" (paper presented at the Society for Maternal-Fetal Medicine Annual Meeting, Grapevine, Texas, February 3–8, 2020). Full manuscript in peer review at the time of publication.

6. B. Spiegel, G. Fuller, M. Lopez, et al., "Virtual Reality for Management of Pain in Hospitalized Patients: A Randomized Comparative Effectiveness Trial," *PLoS ONE* 14 (2019): e0219115.

7. "What Is Precision Medicine?," Genetics Home Reference, January 21, 2020, https://ghr.nlm.nih.gov/primer/precisionmedicine/definition.

8. Pastor Kelvin Sauls recounts the story of So-HELP and discusses "VR-TIME" in his lecture, "So-HELP Me God: How VR Helped Reduce Blood Pressure in the Holman United Methodist Church," 2018 Virtual Medicine Conference at Cedars-Sinai, filmed in Los Angeles, California, with written permission, March 29, 2018, www.youtube.com/watch?v=hZjZuMLkTng. Saul's quotes are obtained from that presentation together with personal discussions.

9. Dr. Bernice Coleman discusses the So-HELP project and its preliminary results in detail in her lecture, "So-HELP Me God: How VR Helped Reduce Blood Pressure in the Holman United Methodist Church," 2018 Virtual Medicine Conference at Cedars-Sinai, filmed in Los Angeles, California, with written permission, March 29, 2018, www.youtube.com/watch?v=hZjZuMLkTng. Dr. Coleman's quote is obtained from that presentation.

10. Coleman, "So-HELP Me God."

11. Brandon Birckhead, Carine Khalil, Xiaoyu Liu, et al., "Recommendations for Methodology of Virtual Reality Clinical Trials in Health Care by an International Working Group: Iterative Study," *JMIR Mental Health* 31 (2019): e11973.

12. Cannon's story was told by *CBS Evening News* in a report titled "Doctor Uses 21st Century Technique to Tackle High Blood Pressure," February 25, 2018, www.cbsnews.com/video/doctor-uses-21st-century-technique-to-tackle-high-blood-pressure.

Chapter 10: The Empathy Machine

1. S. Seinfeld, J. Arroyo-Palacios, G. Iruretagoyena, et al., "Offenders Become the Victim in Virtual Reality: Impact of Changing Perspective in Domestic Violence," *Nature Scientific Reports* 8 (2018): 2692, www.nature.com/articles/s41598-018-19987-7#MOESM1 (to view the movie, scroll down the article and click "Supplementary movie").

2. A. A. Marsh and R. J. R. Blair, "Deficits in Facial Affect Recognition Among Antisocial Populations: A Meta-Analysis," *Neuroscience Biobehavioral Reviews* 32 (2008): 454; M. E. Kret and B. de Gelder, "When a Smile Becomes a Fist: The Perception of

Facial and Bodily Expressions of Emotion in Violent Offenders," *Experimental Brain Research* 228 (2013): 399–410.

3. Elizabeth Bernstein, "The Future of Therapy: Becoming Someone Else in VR," *Wall Street Journal*, April 16, 2018, www.wsj.com/articles/the-future-of-therapy -becoming-someone-else-in-vr-1523888616. In her article, *WSJ* reporter Elizabeth Bernstein also describes her first-person experience in the domestic violence simulator. Although I wrote my own description before having read Bernstein's, the similarities between our experiences are striking. The article also describes experiences from the Catalonian Justice Department in administering the program since 2012. Bernstein writes, "Compared with a control group of 188 aggressors, 191 aggressors who went through the scenario were less likely to commit acts of domestic violence again."

4. L. Maister, N. Sebanz, G. Knoblich, et al., "Experiencing Ownership over a Dark-Skinned Body Reduces Implicit Racial Bias," *Cognition* 128 (2013): 170–178; T. C. Peck, S. Seinfeld, S. M. Aglioti, et al., "Putting Yourself in the Skin of a Black Avatar Reduces Implicit Racial Bias," *Consciousness and Cognition* 22 (2013): 779–787; D. Banakou, D. H. Parasuram, and M. Slater, "Virtual Embodiment of White People in a Black Virtual Body Leads to a Sustained Reduction in Their Implicit Racial Bias," *Frontiers in Human Neuroscience* 10 (2016): 601; V. Groom, J. N. Bailenson, and C. Nass, "The Influence of Racial Embodiment on Racial Bias in Immersive Virtual Environments," *Social Influence* 4 (2009): 1–18.

5. VR boosts empathy for the homeless: T. Asher, E. Ogle, J. N. Bailenson, et al., "Becoming Homeless: A Human Experience," *ACM SIGGRAPH (2018) Virtual, Augmented, and Mixed Reality*. For maltreated children: C. Hamilton-Giachritsis, D. Banakou, M. Garcia Quiroga, et al., "Reducing Risk and Improving Maternal Perspective-Taking and Empathy Using Virtual Embodiment," *Scientific Reports* 8 (2018): 2975. For Syrian refugees: Gabo Arora and Chris Milk, *Clouds over Sidra* (Within, 2015), 360° video, 8:35, http://with.in/watch/clouds-over-sidra. For the elderly: S. Y. Oh, J. N. Bailenson, E. Weisz, et al., "Virtually Old: Embodied Perspective Taking and the Reduction of Ageism Under Threat," *Computers in Human Behavior* 60 (2016): 398–410.

6. Jeremy Bailenson, *Experience on Demand* (New York: W. W. Norton, 2018), 102–106.

7. Bailenson, *Experience on Demand*, 126–130.

8. Mary Chapman, "New Virtual Reality Immersive Lab Embodies Parkinson's, LBD Patients," *Parkinson's News Today*, June 6, 2019, https://parkinsonsnewstoday .com/2019/06/06/new-virtual-reality-immersive-lab-embodies-parkinsons-lbd -patients.

9. There are now hundreds of studies evaluating the impact of VR on learning outcomes in healthcare. Here are just a few, focusing on randomized, controlled trials: A. Foster, N. Chaudhary, K. Thomas, et al., "Using Virtual Patients to Teach Empathy: A Randomized Controlled Study to Enhance Medical Students' Empathic Communication," *Simulation in Healthcare* 11, no. 3 (2016): 181–189; E. Ryan and C. Poole, "Impact of Virtual Learning Environment on Students' Satisfaction, Engagement, Recall, and Retention," *Journal of Medical Imaging Radiation Sciences* (2019): 408–415; C. Ekstrand, A. Jamal, R. Nguyen, et al., "Immersive and Interactive Virtual Reality to Improve

Learning and Retention of Neuroanatomy in Medical Students: A Randomized Controlled Study," *CMAJ Open* 6 (2018): E103–E109; A. Richardson, L. Bracegirdle, S. I. McLachlan, et al., "Use of a Three-Dimensional Virtual Environment to Teach Drug Receptor Interactions," *American Journal of Pharmaceutical Education* (2013): 11.

10. B. Jin, Z. Ai, and and M. Rasmussen, "Simulation of Eye Disease in Virtual Reality," *Conference Proceedings: IEEE Engineering in Medicine and Biology Society* 5 (2005): 5128–5131; Ilyse Liffreing, "Exedrin Is Using Virtual Reality to Show What Having Migraines Are Like," *Digiday*, September 6, 2017, https://digiday.com/marketing/excedrin-using-virtual-reality-show-migraines-like; M. Taubert, L. Webber, T. Hamilton, et al., "Virtual Reality Videos Used in Undergraduate Palliative and Oncology Medical Teaching: Results of a Pilot Study," *BMJ Supportive & Palliative Care* (2019); W. Bunn and J. Terpstra, "Cultivating Empathy for the Mentally Ill Using Simulated Auditory Hallucinations," *Academic Psychiatry* 33 (2009): 457–460; R. K. J. Brown, S. Petty, S. O'Malley, et al., "Virtual Reality Tool Simulates MRI Experience," *Tomography* 4 (2018): 95–98.

11. X. Pan, M. Slater, A. Beacco, et al., "The Responses of Medical General Practitioners to Unreasonable Patient Demand for Antibiotics—A Study of Medical Ethics Using Immersive Virtual Reality," *PLoS ONE* 11 (2016): e0146837.

12. B. O'Sullivan, F. Alam, and C. Matava, "Creating Low-Cost 360-Degree Virtual Reality Videos for Hospitals: A Technical Paper on the Dos and Don'ts," *Journal of Medical Internet Research* 20 (2018): e239.

13. K. Bekelis, D. Calnan, N. Simmons, et al., "Effect of an Immersive Preoperative Virtual Reality Experience on Patient Reported Outcomes: A Randomized Controlled Trial," *Annals of Surgery* 265 (2017): 1068–1073.

14. Carrie Shaw, "The Intersection of VR Storytelling and Healthcare Training," lecture recorded July 16, 2018, Augmented World Expo, www.youtube.com/watch?v=5OCO9oVh4ts.

15. E. Dyer, B. J. Swartzlander, and M. R. Gugliucci, "Using Virtual Reality in Medical Education to Teach Empathy," *Journal of the Medical Library Association* 106 (2018): 498–500.

16. O. Liran, R. Dasher, and K. Kaeochinda, "Using Virtual Reality to Improve Antiretroviral Therapy Adherence in the Treatment of HIV: Open-Label Repeated Measure Study," *Interactive Journal of Medical Research* 8 (2019): e13698.

17. M. Cavazza, G. Aranyi, F. Charles, et al., "Towards Empathic Neurofeedback for Interactive Storytelling," Proceedings of 2014 Workshop on Computational Models of Narrative (CMN 2014), (Quebec City, 2014).

18. J. A. Coan and J. J. B. Allen, "Frontal EEG Asymmetry as a Moderator and Mediator of Emotion," *Biological Psychology* 67 (2004): 7–50.

19. F. Schoeller, P. Bertrand, L. J. Gerry, et al., "Combining Virtual Reality and Biofeedback to Foster Empathic Abilities in Humans," *Frontiers in Psychology* 9 (2019): 2741.

20. For more on triggers of goose bumps and their neurophysiological significance, see these references: M. Benedek and C. Kaernbach, "Physiological Correlates and Emotional Specificity of Human Piloerection," *Biological Psychology* 86 (2011): 320–329; M. Colver and A. El-Alayli, "Getting Aesthetic Chills from Music: The Connection Between Openness to Experience and Frisson," *Psychology of Music* 44 (2016): 413–427;

O. Grewe, R. Kopiez, and E. Altenmüüller, "The Chill Parameter: Goose Bumps and Shivers as Promising Measures in Emotion Research," *Music Perception* 27 (2009): 61–74.

21. D. Quesnel and B. E. Riecke, "Are You Awed Yet? How Virtual Reality Gives Us Awe and Goose Bumps," *Frontiers in Psychology* 9 (2018): 2158.

22. Jessica Hullinger, "The Transcendental Revelations of Astronauts," *The Week*, April 28, 2016, https://theweek.com/articles/619451/transcendental-revelations -astronauts. In the article, NASA astronaut Kathryn Sullivan describes that when she peered out the window of the Soyuz space capsule, she "saw the beautiful blue and white of the Earth below, and the curvature of the horizon. Getting to experience the whole disk of the Earth from that point of view," she said, "was this breathtaking experience. I got goose bumps."

23. Schoeller et al., "Combining Virtual Reality and Biofeedback."

24. Eric Topol, *Deep Medicine: How Artificial Intelligence Can Make Healthcare Human Again* (New York: Basic Books, 2019), 18.

25. There is a burgeoning literature evaluating the negative impact of the electronic health record on physician productivity and well-being. This study revealed slightly more time spent staring at computer screens than meeting with patients (although the title of the paper indicates time is split evenly, there was a tiny edge in favor of desktop charting, and trends only seem to be getting worse): M. Tai-Seale, C. W. Olson, J. Li, et al., "Electronic Health Record Logs Indicate That Physicians Split Time Evenly Between Seeing Patients and Desktop Medicine," *HealthAffairs* (Millwood) 36 (2017): 655–662. Here is another study where the mismatch was greater and in favor of computer time over in-person consultation: L. Block, R. Habicht, A. W. Wu, et al., "In the Wake of the 2003 and 2011 Duty Hours Regulations, How Do Internal Medicine Interns Spend Their Time?," *Journal of General Internal Medicine* 28 (2013): 1042–1047. This study evaluated the impact of algorithmic messages inundating physician inboxes and revealed how it is leading to doctor burnout: M. Tai-Seale, E. C. Dillon, Y. Yang, et al., "Physicians' Well-Being Linked to In-Basket Messages Generated by Algorithms in Electronic Health Records," *HealthAffairs* (Millwood) 38 (2019): 1073–1078.

Chapter 11: Through the Looking Glass

1. "Comparing Two Ways to Help Patients and Doctors Discuss Treatment for Long-Term Pain: Voices in Pain Care," Patient Centered Outcomes Research Institute (PCORI), grant, www.pcori.org/research-results/2016/comparing -two-ways-help-patients-and-doctors-discuss-treatment-long-term-pain.

2. I invented *AbStats* together with Professor William Kaiser in the School of Engineering at UCLA. The device was FDA cleared in 2015. We validated its use in these studies: M. Kaneshiro, W. Kaiser, J. Pourmorady, et al., "Postoperative Gastrointestinal Telemetry with an Acoustic Biosensor Predicts Ileus vs. Uneventful GI Recovery," *Journal of Gastrointestinal Surgery* 20 (2016): 132–139; B. M. Spiegel, M. Kaneshiro, M. M. Russell, et al., "Validation of an Acoustic Gastrointestinal Surveillance Biosensor for Postoperative Ileus," *Journal of Gastrointestinal Surgery* 10 (2014): 1795–1803.

3. A. D. Deemer, C. K. Bradley, N. C. Ross, et al., "Low Vision Enhancement with Head-Mounted Video Display Systems: Are We There Yet?," *Optometry and Vision Science* 9 (2018): 694–703.

4. "Goggles 'Give Back' Sight to Maisy so She Can Read Again," BBC News, June 10, 2019, www.bbc.com/news/av/technology-48501600/goggles-give -back-sight-to-maisy-so-she-can-read-again.

5. Mary Kekatos, "Hope for Millions with Vision Loss: Virtual Reality Headset Allows Legally Blind People to See Their Surroundings and Read," *Daily Mail*, August 2, 2018, www.dailymail.co.uk/health/article-6020245/VR-headset-help-restore -eye-sight-macular-degeneration.html.

6. A. D. Deemer, B. K. Swenor, K. Fujiwara, et al., "Preliminary Evaluation of Two Digital Image Processing Strategies for Head-Mounted Magnification for Low Vision Patients," *Translational Vision Science and Technology* 8 (2019): 23.

7. K. E. Laver, B. Lange, S. George, et al., "Virtual Reality for Stroke Rehabilitation," *Cochrane Database of Systematic Reviews* 20 (2017): CD008349.

8. Dave Muoio, "FDA Clears MindMaze's Gamified Home-Neurorehabilitation Platform," *MobiHealthNews*, June 12, 2018, www.mobihealthnews.com/content /fda-clears-mindmazes-gamified-home-neurorehabilitation-platform. For more information about MindMaze visit www.mindmaze.com.

9. Richard Bashara, "Why Your Brain May Be Hardwired for VR Fitness," VR Fitness Insider, May 6, 2019, www.vrfitnessinsider.com/why-your-brain-may -be-hardwired-for-vr-fitness.

10. For more on Black Box VR, visit www.blackbox-vr.com.

11. M. S. Kamińska, A. Miller, I. Rotter, et al., "The Effectiveness of Virtual Reality Training in Reducing the Risk of Falls Among Elderly People," *Clinical Interventions in Aging* 13 (2018): 2329–2338.

12. L. I. Gómez-Jordana, J. Stafford, C. L. E. Peper, et al., "Virtual Footprints Can Improve Walking Performance in People with Parkinson's Disease," *Frontiers in Neurology* 9 (2018): 681.

13. M. Matsangidou, C. Ang, A. R. Mauger, et al., "Is Your Virtual Self as Sensational as Your Real? Virtual Reality: The Effect of Body Consciousness on the Experience of Exercise Sensations," *Psychology of Sport and Exercise* 41 (2019): 218–224.

14. For more on Karuna Labs, visit www.karunavr.com.

15. A. R. Donati, S. Shokur, E. Morya, et al., "Long-Term Training with a Brain-Machine Interface-Based Gait Protocol Induces Partial Neurological Recovery in Paraplegic Patients," *Scientific Reports* 6 (2016): 30383.

16. S. Zhang, Q. Fu, S. Guo, et al., "Coordinative Motion-Based Bilateral Rehabilitation Training System with Exoskeleton and Haptic Devices for Biomedical Application," *Micromachines* (Basel) 10 (2018).

17. A. Rizzo, G. Lucas, J. Gratch, et al., "Automatic Behavior Analysis During a Clinical Interview with a Virtual Human," *Studies in Health Technology and Informatics* 220 (2016): 316–322, PubMed PMID: 27046598.

18. J. Marín-Morales, J. L. Higuera-Trujillo, A. Greco, et al., "Affective Computing in Virtual Reality: Emotion Recognition from Brain and Heartbeat Dynamics Using Wearable Sensors," *Scientific Reports* 8 (2018): 13657.

19. VR is now being used by a growing number of preeminent medical schools. Here is information about the VR program at New York University: NYU Langone Health, "Virtual and Augmented Reality," https://med.nyu.edu/departments

-institutes/innovations-medical-education/education-technology/virtual-augmented
-reality. Information about the VR program at the University of California, San Francisco: Mitzi Baker, "How VR Is Revolutionizing the Way Future Doctors Are Learning About Our Bodies," UCSF, September 18, 2017, www.ucsf.edu/news/2017/09/408301/how-vr-revolutionizing-way-future-doctors-are-learning-about-our-bodies.

20. G. Blumstein, B. Jukotynski, N. Cevallos, et al., "Tibial IMN: Virtual Reality vs. Standard Surgical Guide—A Randomized Study," Western Orthopaedic Association Annual Meeting, 2019, Monterey, California.

21. S. D. Delshad, C. V. Almario, G. Fuller, et al., "Economic Analysis of Implementing Virtual Reality Therapy for Pain Among Hospitalized Patients," *NPJ Digital Medicine* 1 (2018): 22.

22. Walt Disney Company, "Disney Team of Heroes Debuts Innovative Experiences at Texas Children's Hospital," press release, April 17, 2019, www.thewaltdisneycompany.com/disney-team-of-heroes-debuts-innovative-experiences-at-texas-childrens-hospital.

23. Robert Wachter, *The Digital Doctor: Hope, Hype, and Harm at the Dawn of Medicine's Computer Age* (New York: McGraw-Hill, 2015). In this exceptional book, UCSF Chairman of Medicine Bob Wachter describes the hope, hype, and harm at the dawn of medicine's computer age. He offers examples where digital technologies can help improve patient outcomes, but also illustrates how computers can mislead doctors, arrive at false conclusions, undermine the patient-doctor relationship, and cause terrible yet preventable outcomes.

Index

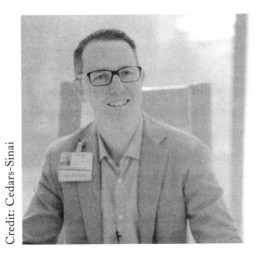

Brennan Spiegel is Director of Health-Services Research at Cedars-Sinai Medical Center and Professor of Medicine and Public Health at the University of California, Los Angeles. Dr. Spiegel directs the Cedars-Sinai Center for Outcomes Research and Education, a multidisciplinary team that investigates how technology can strengthen the patient-doctor bond and improve clinical outcomes. His team developed one of the largest and most widely documented therapeutic virtual reality programs in the world at Cedars-Sinai. He founded Virtual Medicine, an international symposium dedicated to medical virtual reality. He lives in Los Angeles, California. For the latest on Dr. Spiegel's research, you can follow him on Twitter @BrennanSpiegel and online at www.virtualmedicine.health/blog.